"The authors of *Animal Reiki* have demystified their subject in an objective and clear way, rendering this much-neglected healing art more accessible to readers and, more importantly, to our wonderful animal friends."

—CHRISTOPHER DAY, MA, VetMB, VetFFHom, MRCVS
author of *Homoeopathic Treatment of Small Animals: Principles and Practice*

"*Animal Reiki* is a great introduction to the growing field of energy medicine. Written in an easy-to-read style, this book will be enjoyed by animal guardians and veterinarians alike. Anyone who wants to learn about holistic therapy can now add another modality to the list of possible treatments."

—SHAWN MESSONNIER, DVM
host of *Dr. Shawn—The Natural Vet* on Martha Stewart Radio (Sirius) and author of the award-winning *The Natural Health Bible for Dogs & Cats*

"This beautiful introduction to healing animals with Reiki speaks a language of love and light that knows no species boundary. The format is thorough enough for the professional yet accessible to all. Compassion flows from every page."

—SHARON CALLAHAN, Animal Communication Specialist
author of *Healing Animals Naturally*

"What a wonderful gift Elizabeth Fulton and Kathleen Prasad have given to humans and in turn the animals of the world. This inspirational work takes the mystery out of Reiki, thereby empowering animal lovers to offer unconditional love, understanding and healing to the animals who have given us so much."

—LISA ROSS-WILLIAMS
host of the *If Your Horse Could Talk* show

"*Animal Reiki* is an excellent resource for everyone interested in healing animals. This book is a powerful reminder of the wider uses of the system of Reiki and how humanity can be of purposeful benefit to all."

—BRONWEN AND FRANS STIENE, International House of Reiki
authors of *A-Z of Reiki*, *The Japanese Art of Reiki* and *The Reiki Sourcebook*

Animal Reiki

using energy to heal the animals in your life

Elizabeth Fulton
Kathleen Prasad

Foreword by **Cheryl Schwartz, DVM**
Photography by **Kendra Luck**

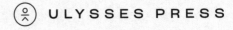 **ULYSSES PRESS**

Published by: Ulysses Press
P.O. Box 3440
Berkeley, CA 94703
www.ulyssespress.com

ISBN: 978-1-56975-528-0
Library of Congress Control Number: 2005908369

Printed in Canada by Marquis Book Printing

20 19 18 17 16 15 14 13

Editorial and production staff: Lily Chou, Claire Chun, Matt Orendorff,
    Steven Schwartz
Acquisitions Editor: Ashley Chase
Index: Sayre Van Young
Design: Lourdes Robles
Cover photography: front cover: Pets & Vets disc © jupiterimages.com;
    back cover: Kendra Luck
Interior photography: Kendra Luck except pages 15, 31, 49, 62, 65, 70, 72, 142, 144, 201, 219 courtesy of Elizabeth Fulton; pages 54, 61, 141, 149, 150, 151 courtesy of Jamie Westdal; pages 30, 53, 213 courtesy of Earl McCowen; page 109 courtesy of Delphine Hano; page 176 courtesy of Carol Buckley of The Elephant Sanctuary; page 233 courtesy of Susanna Anthony

For Bob and Laura

—Elizabeth Fulton

For my dearest Che

—Kathleen Prasad

Table of Contents

Foreword *by Cheryl Schwartz, DVM*

ANIMALS ARE THE GREATEST TEACHERS. Without being overbearing or pedantic, they seem to show us ways of progressing on our paths with kindness, strength and humor. It's only fitting that we reciprocate in kind. The Reiki healing system is perfect for this as it carries with it respectful acknowledgement of animals' expansive capabilities. Masters of energetic integration, animals intuitively understand that we all exist on physical, emotional, mental and spiritual levels simultaneously. With this understanding, they are naturals at accepting Reiki into their lives.

Being a holistic veterinarian and healer for over 25 years, I have participated in the wave of energy healing, being privy to inexplicable and wonderful animal recoveries similar to those recounted in this book. Whether I am utilizing Chinese medicine, acupuncture, herbs, homeopathy or flower essences, I am convinced that energy medicine is both the momentum of the future and the core of tradition.

Reiki is a complete energy healing system that invites connection with the Universal Source, asking us to tap into its vast consciousness with respect and reverence. In this book, Elizabeth Fulton and Kathleen Prasad take us on a Reiki journey, showing how Reiki goes to the center of a problem, considers the whole being, and gently orchestrates a healing process.

Many of my clients have told me of the miraculous help Reiki has been for their animal companions. Although I have been duly impressed, I have never formally studied the system, never making the time to take the classes. Thus I was thrilled to hear this book was coming out to explain Reiki more fully.

Animals have always assured me that using intuition (itself communication with the Universal Source) is an effective tool for treating and re-balancing health. Intuition is based upon trust, another element the animals teach. This book shows us countless examples of trust, exhibited both by the authors in their practice and their animal recipients. Each animal patient is respectfully offered Reiki and given freedom of choice for acceptance.

Intuitively I have been working with energy fields surrounding my patients' bodies to diagnose and treat disorders, frequently experiencing sensations of heat, cold, texture or tingling at precisely the location of imbalance. As my palm scans specific areas above the animal's body, I have been given pictures or scenes from earlier times in the animal's life, or experience emotional sensations.

From this, I have learned that many of our animal companions' chronic physical problems really are preceded by emotional trauma that has not been fully resolved. Recognizing the energetic existence of the imbalance is the prelude to healing. It was gratifying to read in this book that my experience is similar to what is described as Reiki, and yet it has been the animals who have taught it to me: a prime example of how healing is offered by the universe to everyone.

One cat, Chloe, came to see me. She was plagued by chronic stiffness and intermittent lameness in her hind end, ongoing for several years. Although Chloe's human had been to several vets and Chloe had done all the tests, still no cause or treatment abated the problem. Acupuncture had given temporary relief, but now Chloe was miserable, not wanting to jump up or go outside.

When I examined Chloe by scanning the energy about six inches above her spine, I came to a specific area towards the base of her spine and my hand just stopped mid-air. It didn't want to move. I felt nauseated, outraged and sad all at once. So while holding my palm above this area, I asked if Chloe had ever been injured there. The woman shook her head no, but then, still thinking, she remembered that when Chloe was a young cat she had been attacked by a neighborhood cat bully and bitten right there. An abscess formed, but it was lanced, and Chloe was given antibiotics. All was healed.

The stiffness began one year after that time, and now two years later I was finding a bundle of emotions stuck in the energy field above her body at the exact place where she had been bitten. Just by recognizing and remembering this incident and sharing the emotions involved, the energy block began to dissipate. Chloe began the healing process. After several more "treatments," she recovered and is now running like she was a kitten.

Little did I know that part of my treatment was very similar to what is described in this book as Reiki! Throughout the book, I have been repeatedly impressed by Ms. Fulton's and Prasad's respect for all animals' integrity, and by the authors' understanding of including the animal in his treatment by asking his permission *before doing something to him*, a far cry from usual medical behavior.

I was so in tune with this book that it could have been me writing it, recounting stories. No wonder the universe sent me that email asking if I would write the foreword. Thank you, Elizabeth and Kathleen, for writing this book. Animal lovers will totally appreciate it and hopefully use what it has to offer.

This book has been written from the Heart and to the Heart. The Reiki jumps off the pages, giving a healing to the reader. Any of you who are intuitive will feel it and let it open your heart even more.

Authors' Preface

TRADITIONALLY, REIKI PRACTICE and teaching have centered on healing humans. However, there are many reasons why we have chosen to focus the practice of Reiki on the animal kingdom. We believe animals are sentient, spiritual beings who give generously of themselves to the planet and are innately deserving of Reiki's benefits.

Living with people and civilization exacts a great toll on animals. They are often deprived of their natural habitats, freedom and ability to manifest their full natures, sexuality and reproductive function, yet they continue to show us devotion, loyalty and an amazing capacity for forgiveness. They are often misunderstood, and the enormous gifts they offer mankind are not recognized or honored. They cannot speak their needs and wants in human terms and are often dependent upon people for the satisfaction of even their most basic needs.

Animals teach us many things. They teach us to listen, to live in the moment, to forgive and to be joyful. Animals teach us about commitment and acceptance. They are our confidantes and comforters. They also have a way of bringing up our own issues so that we must deal with them and, in the process, grow. For many of us, our most profound experiences of unconditional love have been with an animal. And many offer us extraordinary gifts as working animals: guide dogs, therapy horses, search-and-rescue and other service animals. Because of domestic animals' close contact and bond with humans, they often internalize and reflect their people's problems. This sympathetic connection can manifest as a problem for the animal on the physical, emotional or spiritual level.

■ How Reiki can help animals heal

Reiki can help animals in myriad ways. Practicing Reiki with your animal companion deepens your bond as well as the level of understanding and trust between you. With healthy animals, Reiki can help maintain health on all levels. Reiki can heal physical illness and injury in animals as well as problems on emotional and spiritual levels. It is a powerful tool for emotional healing following trauma, abuse, neglect, fear and trust issues, reaching deeply into even the most damaged spirits.

For high-strung or nervous animals, Reiki induces deep relaxation and stress-reduction and, over time, can reduce the tendency toward nervousness. Reiki can accelerate healing after surgery or illness. It complements both conventional and alternative therapies and can enhance their actions and lessen their side effects. Finally, for a dying animal and his people, Reiki provides compassionate support that can make the transition more peaceful for all concerned.

■ Why Reiki is ideal for healing animals

Although Reiki traditionally has been used primarily for humans, it has many qualities that make it an ideal complementary therapy for animals. First and foremost, it is gentle, painless, non-invasive

and stress-free for animals. Reiki heals at all levels of an animal's being: physical, mental, emotional and spiritual. It is one of only a few therapies that brings no harm to any living thing—plant or animal—to produce its healing properties. It goes to those issues most in need of healing, even those unknown to the practitioner.

Reiki is always safe and comfortable for both animal and healer. It can be given at a distance and adapted to any problem that affects animals, so it can be used under any circumstances. There is virtually no problem or circumstance that cannot be treated effectively with Reiki.

Although it is powerful and always goes to the source of health problems, Reiki can do no harm to the recipient or the practitioner. Reiki is a simple method that can heal complex problems. There is a deep sense of gratitude on both sides after a treatment.

■ Creating a powerful healing partnership

With Reiki, animals do not have to be confined or restrained to be treated. The Reiki practitioner works with the animal to deter-

THE WAITING STAG

One day as I was coming in from the car carrying groceries, I encountered a deer in our entry courtyard. It is not unusual to find deer there. The herd that lives in my neighborhood knows that I am fond of them and that they are safe here. But this deer, a young stag who had just shed his antlers, was unfamiliar to me, and he was standing there with a very purposeful expression on his face, as though he had been waiting for me.

He looked directly at me and held up his left rear leg. When I didn't immediately comprehend his message, he turned around and licked the area above his hind hoof several times. Sure enough, there was a half-dollar-size chunk of flesh missing, with a deep puncture in the middle of the wound, and the area was red, swollen and infected. From the pronounced limp he showed when he took a couple of steps, I could tell it was extremely painful.

I put my groceries in the kitchen, sat down on the doorstep and offered him Reiki. Almost immediately I felt a strong flow of Reiki energy. The young stag stood facing me for a while, then shifted so that the injured leg was the part of his body closest to me. Gradually his head lowered and his eyes half-

mine how the treatment will be given. The animal retains a large degree of control over his own process of healing, including how much Reiki he will take and under what circumstances, so that he becomes an active and willing partner in the healing process.

Reiki is a vibrational "frequency" that is readily understood and appreciated by an animal, allowing him to deepen his relationship with the practitioner as he joins in a healing partnership. With repeated treatments, animals come to seek Reiki out on their own when they need relaxation or healing.

Over time Reiki also deepens the healer's intuition and enables her to communicate at a deeper level with her animal clients, building a high level of intimacy and trust between human healer and animal recipient. Reiki healing becomes a profoundly rewarding experience for both human and animal.

For both partners in the healing process, Reiki transforms the understanding of what is possible within the human/animal relationship. In this way, Reiki brings healing not only to individual animals and people, but also to the human/animal bond, thus

closed as he relaxed into a semi-dozing "Reiki state," the injured leg twitching occasionally.

It was a chilly day, and only a small patch of sun shone into the entry courtyard. Several times during the treatment the stag roused himself from his half-dozing state and moved over to the patch of sunlight as it shifted around the courtyard, carefully positioning his injured leg closest to me each time. This continued for an hour, at which point I had to end the treatment because of an appointment. I was honored that this young deer had come to me for healing.

The next day I found him waiting for me—twice! Each time I was able to put everything aside and sit down and offer him Reiki. During the first treatment, some neighborhood dogs started barking menacingly nearby and he bounded off, but several hours later he was back, ready to resume his treatment. Each time his head went down and he entered a relaxed "Reiki state" more quickly than he had the previous treatment. The deer came for daily treatments for the next several weeks, missing only days when there were heavy rains or carpenters at work in the courtyard. A month later his wound had healed and his limp had disappeared, but he continued to come for short treatments every few days, apparently greatly enjoying the experience of a Reiki treatment and understanding its healing action.—*Elizabeth*

healing the interconnectedness of all living beings.

▬ Who can benefit from learning Reiki with animals?

The ability to heal with Reiki energy can be easily acquired by anyone with an interest in healing animals and deepening her relationship with animals. For people who live with animal companions, Reiki is a wonderful gift to offer them. Reiki is also an invaluable skill for people who work professionally with animals.

For example, dog groomers, dog trainers, vet technicians, animal acupressure and massage therapists, TTouch practitioners, shelter and sanctuary staff and volunteers, animal rescue specialists, wildlife rehabilitators, horse trainers of all disciplines, chiropractors, veterinarians and animal communicators have found Reiki to be a worthwhile adjunct to the services they offer to animals.

Reiki is representative of an energetic approach to healing that is underutilized in our culture and adds an important dimension to the healing available to animals in our society.

There are other powerful energetic healing modalities available to animals, but the potential of Reiki for healing animals has not yet been fully explored. By outlining the benefits of the Reiki healing system, we hope to increase awareness of the benefits of Reiki and of energy healing for animals in general. By making the fullest possible range of healing options available to animals, we can heal our bond with them and, in the process, our own souls as well.

■ Basic Reiki can be learned easily and quickly

Becoming a Reiki practitioner does not require any special skills, inherent healing ability or spiritual beliefs. The key to becoming a Reiki healer is not years of study, reading and memorization but taking the knowledge and Reiki energy received in a class and then practicing on your own, asking questions as they arise.

This does not mean Reiki is a minor healing art or a curiosity to be mastered in a weekend. It is a powerful healing tool that came to the West from Japan and is passed on from Master to student. By receiving energy attunements (also called initiations) and some basic teachings from a Reiki Master, anyone with a desire to learn can become a Reiki healer.

Reiki begins to heal through the practitioner immediately after the attunements, but the practitioner's understanding of healing grows and deepens with time and practice. Energetic in essence, Reiki can be practiced successfully in combination with any belief system and background. The understanding of Reiki unfolds continually as the practitioner uses Reiki, observes what happens and asks questions, if necessary.

It is sometimes said that "Reiki teaches Reiki," because as a practitioner uses Reiki, the understanding of its nature and potential naturally unfolds. Part of its simple beauty is that it is immediately accessible and effective for the beginner but involves many levels of understanding. Even the most experienced practitioners continue to learn as they practice.

For those who choose to practice Reiki with animals, the animals also become important teachers, guiding practitioners to greater understanding of healing and showing them how to give the most suitable treatment to each individual.

■ Our goal in writing this book

The aim of this book is to educate people about the many benefits of Reiki as a holistic healing system for animals. We would like to see Reiki become a widely available and commonly used complementary therapy for animals. We have included many stories of our experiences with animals and the lessons we have learned from them. We also have outlined the best strategies for using Reiki with animals that we have learned from our animal teachers. We hope our experiences and suggestions will provide a starting point for you to begin to offer Reiki healing to the animals in your life, and we hope you share our excitement as you join us in our journey into the largely unexplored field of animal Reiki. As The Waiting Stag story on page xiv indicates, the animals are, quite literally, waiting for you.

An Introduction to Reiki

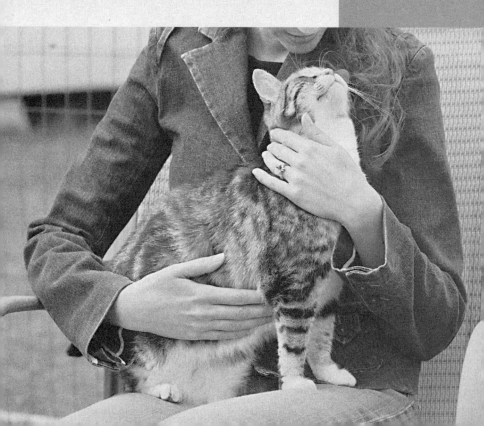

chapter 1

A Basic Understanding of Reiki

AS WE BEGIN discussing Reiki with animals, we'd like to give a brief introduction to Reiki in general. We hope this background will provide a cornerstone of shared understanding for the rest of the book.

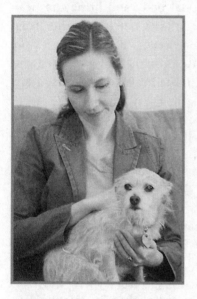

Today, there are many schools of Reiki, but all of these schools originated with the founder of Reiki, Dr. Mikao Usui. In all schools, Reiki is passed on from Master to student through initiations, as Dr. Usui practiced. Although the student receives a basic understanding of Reiki from her Master, personal practice results in unique, individual interpretations, healing experiences and personal growth. We celebrate the fact that all schools of Reiki, despite their differences, spread the healing gift of Reiki throughout the world.

■■ What is Reiki and what does it do?

The term "Reiki" is usually translated as "universal life energy." It is a holistic healing system, meaning that it treats the whole being, addressing problems and healing at all levels: physical, mental, emotional and spiritual. Along with other therapies, such as acupuncture, homeopathy, Qi Gong and flower essence therapy, Reiki is part of the emerging field of energetic healing, rediscovered from the wisdom and knowledge of ancient cultures for use in modern times. Everything in the universe is made up of and connected by energy. By transmitting the healing energy of the universe along energetic pathways and through the practitioner's hands to the client, Reiki heals as deeply as needed within a being to create a shift toward health.

A Reiki treatment can be given in person, with the hands of the practitioner placed on or at a short distance from the client; or, since Reiki is energetic in essence, it can be sent across a distance, across a room or to another geographic location. Reiki can be used to maintain health and energetic balance in a healthy being, to heal illness, injuries, emotional and spiritual problems, and to ease the transition between life and death.

Reiki goes directly to the source of the problem, even if it's unknown to practitioner and client, and heals at a level and intensity that a being is open to receive. If the healing that's most necessary involves some aspect of his situation, Reiki will go beyond the being's physical and emotional body and bring the healing that's needed to the situation. Reiki will benefit not only the animals being treated but also the health of the person giving it. Every time a Reiki practitioner gives a treatment, the Reiki flows through her, healing

THE CAT WHO KNEW WHAT HE NEEDED

Carlton was an unusually large and very beautiful six-month-old cat. He had come from a breeder who kept a large number of cats in her basement and gave them little attention. His limited contact with people had been primarily around unpleasant events, like going to the vet for vaccinations. His person Jenny loved him but was easily hurt by the distance he kept from her, which she saw as his refusal to give her a chance. By the time she called me, the situation between them had grown quite tense, and Jenny was considering taking Carlton back to the breeder.

When I arrived for the treatment, I said hello to Carlton, sat down on the floor in the middle of the living room, and explained who I was, why I was there, and asked him to take only what he wanted in the way of energy. Just as he decided to dash from under the table, across the room and behind the couch, I put my hands out and began the treatment. In mid-dash he jumped as though startled, became still, and looked long and hard at me. Then he sprinted over, stood on my lap with his paws on my shoulder, and licked my face. He looked directly and curiously into my eyes for a moment, and then finished his dash to behind the couch. It was as though he had said, "I'm so glad you're here! Boy, do we need you!" Jenny was speechless since he had never done anything like that before and had always kept a safe distance from people.

her and the client simultaneously. The feeling of receiving a Reiki treatment is generally one of deep relaxation.

Over time Reiki deepens your intuition, so that a deeper level of communication with your animal becomes possible. As you practice Reiki and receive Reiki treatments, it brings out who you are at the most authentic level, enhancing your innate gifts, talents and potential. In practicing Reiki with animals, you'll find that the more animals you treat, the more you'll encounter animals who need healing. Animals understand Reiki's benefits and will seek you out when they need healing. The beauty of Reiki as a healing system is its simple, gentle nature combined with its powerful and transformative results.

▬ Learning Reiki

Anyone can learn to practice Reiki. The length and format of Beginning (Level 1) Reiki classes vary from Reiki Master to Reiki Master. The most common formats involve six to ten hours of instruction over a period of two

For a while Carlton moved around the room from hiding place to hiding place, although I could feel from the flow of energy in my hands that he was choosing to accept the treatment. Finally he stretched himself out on the floor about three feet away and, with a huge sigh, put his head on his paws and went to sleep. He slept for 20 minutes or so, got up, looked quite intensely at me, and then went on about his business, indicating that the treatment was over. As I left, he ran up to my side for a moment before dashing out of sight.

Carlton had six treatments and, from the first, things began to improve. He began to sleep next to Jenny some nights and to join her on the couch when she watched TV. Jenny realized that she needed to be patient with him, and that his wariness was not related to his feelings about her personally, but was learned in his former environment. In the end, they were able to reach a compromise that made them both happy. Jenny accepted that Carlton would never be the kind of cat she could just scoop up and cuddle anytime she wanted, and Carlton understood that he really was loved and safe and began to seek her out when he was in the mood for affection. —*Elizabeth*

to four days; the classes include basic instruction in what Reiki is, its history and principles, and how it's used for self-treatment and the treatment of others. Also included are four energy attunements that enable Reiki energy to begin to flow from the student's hands. Some people can feel Reiki energy flowing through their hands immediately; for others, it takes some time and practice to be able to feel the energy flow. Whether or not the student can feel the flow of energy, Reiki begins to heal through her as soon as she receives the Reiki attunements.

THE REIKI ATTUNEMENTS

An attunement (or initiation, as it is also called) is the Master-to-student transference of the ability to use Reiki energy for healing. It involves a series of sacred steps passed down from Reiki Master to Reiki Master. During or soon after the initiations, students sometimes feel energetic sensations such as heat or an ache on the crown of the head, light-headedness, or pressure or heat in the palms of the hands. These sensations are short-lived and disappear as the energy is assimilated into the student's system. Traditionally, initiations are

THE LITTLE DOG WHO RECOGNIZED REIKI

Sometimes animals can recognize and be drawn to Reiki's healing energy even without a treatment. In the early days of my animal Reiki experiences, I decided to visit an animal sanctuary. As I was walking through the "intake" kennels, where dogs were first brought in, one of the employees came in and explained the history of the various dogs to me. Then she began to tell me about her own dog, whom she brought to work with her each day. This sweet little dog had been found abandoned with a bullet in her head, three broken ribs, an open wound, and almost starved to death. They thought she wouldn't survive, but with lots of tender loving care and surgery, she fought the odds and won. However, she still didn't like strangers.

As the employee finished her story, her little dog jumped up on me. I leaned down and she put one paw up on my lap, stretched her little body upward, and solemnly licked my face several times. Her owner was absolutely amazed! She then asked if I was a spiritual person. I shared with her that I was a Reiki practitioner. She replied that she "should have known," because her little dog was an old soul who recognized and was attracted to spiritual energy. Needless to say, I was quite amazed and taken aback. This experience gave me a newfound respect for animals' awareness of energy. —*Kathleen*

spaced out over several hours or days so that the student can adjust more comfortably to the Reiki energy.

LEARNING A NEW "LANGUAGE"

Learning Reiki is much like learning a new language. Energetic sensations are often very subtle and may take some time to learn to recognize. The more you practice Reiki, the more you'll become adept at the language of energy, and the more you'll feel the energy in your hands and perhaps other parts of yourself. At the same time, the feeling in your hands or body doesn't necessarily mirror the power of the treatment. Sometimes you may feel little or nothing, yet the animal will experience a dramatic healing response. Reiki practitioners learn to "trust Reiki" because it is Reiki, not you, that does the healing. With practice, you will learn to recognize the many ways healing can manifest.

Reiki is best learned through practice, questions and observation. Once initiated, a student has immediate and effective access to Reiki energy for life. Reiki's healing results are as accessible to the novice as they are to the expert.

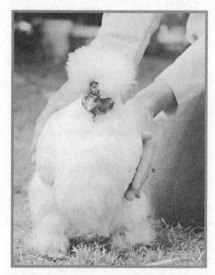

Poodle, a silky chicken, accepts a hands-on Reiki treatment.

You can continue to be challenged by and learn from this practice all your life, but it is a powerful healing tool when practiced by even a beginner. This ability to heal with Reiki will never go away, regardless of how little you practice. However, the more you open yourself up to the practice of Reiki, the more you will understand Reiki's subtle yet powerful nature. The efficacy of a Reiki treatment is determined by the essence of Reiki itself, not by your knowledge. Even after many years of practice, wise practitioners remain humble and always remember to thank Reiki for the results it brings about.

THREE LEVELS OF REIKI PRACTICE

Level 1: Beginning Reiki. This level of practice involves giving self-treatments and treatments to others hands-on or from a short distance away. At this level of Reiki, the practitioner becomes familiar with the nature and use of Reiki, how it feels to be a conduit for Reiki energy, and the healing results Reiki can bring. Because of the complete and effective nature of Reiki at Level 1, many people who practice Reiki with humans choose to remain at this level of Reiki for life. For those who want to practice with animals, however, having Level 2 Reiki greatly expands the circumstances under which you can give treatments to animals.

Level 2: Advanced Reiki. This level of practice involves learning three ancient symbols that can be used to intensify the Reiki

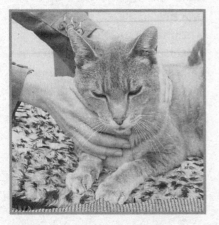

flow, to focus healing on the mental and emotional levels, and to send Reiki across greater distances. Level 2 Reiki is especially useful in working with animals. Since Level 2 Reiki enables you to send treatments to an animal at a safe distance or while out of the animal's presence, it is possible to treat any animal under virtually any circumstances. Wild, aggressive, abused and traumatized animals can be treated safely and comfortably with distant Reiki. They can enter into a relationship to be healed without the necessity of confinement, restraint, unacceptable proximity to a human being, or submitting to human touch.

Mental and emotional healing can be intensified as well with Level 2 Reiki. The powerful nature of Level 2 Reiki enables it to reach deeply into even the most damaged spirits to bring about healing. With Level 2 Reiki, you'll become acquainted with the true range of possibilities for bringing healing to animals. After receiving Level 2 Reiki, most people choose to stay at this level of practice.

Level 3: Becoming a Reiki Master. In our view, becoming a Reiki Master is for the truly dedicated student who is motivated to make a life commitment to the practice of Reiki. At this level the student receives the ability to pass on Reiki to others and thus become a teacher. Also, at this level of Reiki, the flow of energy will be intensified, which will often bring new healing challenges for you in your own life as well as your Reiki practice. Becoming a Reiki Master is not the end of the learning process but the beginning of a new journey in healing and personal growth.

■ Finding a Reiki teacher

Each Reiki student should find the Master Teacher who resonates best with her philosophy and way of being in the world. It is our experience that Reiki is able to find and enhance each person's individual gifts and transform her life in a truly healing way. Our interpretations and suggestions in this book represent our understanding of Reiki. If you have already learned Reiki, we encourage you to take from us what resonates with you and go out and start practicing with animals. If you have not yet learned Reiki, we hope this chapter has given you a starting point for talking with prospective Reiki teachers about Reiki philosophy and practice. It's important that you find a Reiki teacher with whom you feel comfortable, encouraged and supported so that you can receive the best possible foundation for your own unique path as you go out into the world to offer healing to animals.

chapter 2

Overview of a Reiki Treatment

WITH HUMANS, A REIKI treatment is given with the hands of the practitioner on or close to the fully clothed body of the client. An established sequence of specific hand positions (which do not involve touching any private areas of the body) is generally followed out of respect for tradition and because extensive experience has shown that this approach ensures a comprehensive treatment. Most experienced practitioners will diverge from the sequence at times when their intuition suggests that additional positions or changes in the sequence will better provide what is needed for the individual client, but the traditional sequence is the starting point for most people.

■ Adapting treatments for working with animals

When we first began practicing Reiki with animals, we assumed that we should just use this sequence of hands-on positions, with adaptations as necessary to accommodate animals' different sizes, shapes and postures, and the fact that they're not lying on a massage table. Over time the animals themselves showed us that treatments for animals are

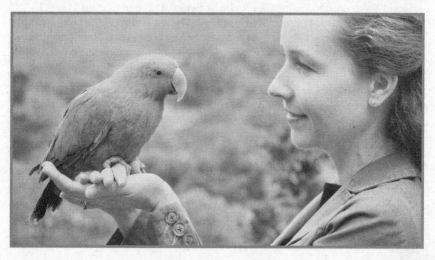

usually best given from at least a short distance. We have found that this is sometimes a hard concept for people trained in Reiki with humans to accept. However, with Reiki, there is no reason why an animal cannot have exactly the treatment that best suits him. We will elaborate on this idea in Part Two, but we encourage people who have been practicing with humans to begin to think outside the box, because, in general, this will serve them well in treating animals with Reiki. One of the most exciting aspects of animal Reiki for us is that no two treatments are exactly alike. Each new animal and circumstance will need something slightly different, so giving Reiki treatments always involves some creativity.

▬ What happens during a treatment?

The duration of a Reiki treatment varies by situation, client and practitioner. Most commonly, hands-on or other in-person treatments for animals as well as people last about one hour. Distant treatments are usually shorter in length. When receiving a Reiki

COMMUNICATING WITH SILENCE

Reiki can reach even the most traumatized cases. One dog that I was treating at the shelter was an incessant barker. She barked and barked, her eyes staring blankly ahead of her. I put in my earplugs and began the treatment from outside her kennel. For the first 20 minutes, she barked nonstop, staring into my face. I suddenly got the intuition that she believed no one listened to her. I mentally told her that I was listening to her. She immediately stopped barking and lay down in the back of the kennel facing away from me. Simultaneously, I had a strong feeling that she'd been tied up in a back yard with no one ever coming out to visit her, except to yell at her for barking.

She remained quiet and restful for about 15 minutes, until a loud crash somewhere else in the shelter snapped her out of it and she resumed her barking. I mentally told her that she didn't have to bark anymore, that she would be listened to now. Her behavior didn't change for the duration of the treatment, and when I left, she was still barking. I wondered about my intuition during the treatment, so as I left the shelter that day, I asked one of the employees what her background was. She said the dog had been tied up outside and neglected. I asked the employee to visit her regularly and tell her each time that she was being listened to. On a subsequent visit, I was happy to see that her barking had decreased significantly. —*Kathleen*

treatment, people and animals commonly enter a state of deep relaxation and peace. They may feel heat, tingling or pulsing. They may sigh, yawn, doze, fall asleep or even enter a deep state of meditation. Some people sense the energetic ebb and flow of the healing energy while others feel little. Some continue to converse with the practitioner throughout the treatment. Regardless of their experience during the treatment, most people and animals notice health improvements afterwards.

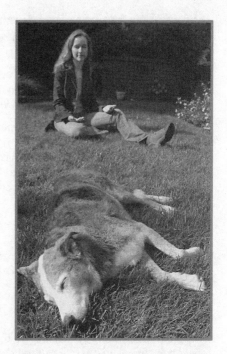

Animals are much more sensitive than humans to energy in general and feel Reiki energy immediately and strongly. Many animals will startle or stop in their tracks when they first feel Reiki energy. They will usually look very intensely at you; domestic animals often will come over and sniff your hands.

How animals react to this new sensation depends upon their temperament and previous experience with humans. They may recognize the healing potential of Reiki immediately, sigh gratefully and settle quickly into a relaxed position to absorb the energy, or, if their experiences with humans have not been positive, they may initially seek to avoid the energy. We'll talk about how to deal with this reaction in the following chapters.

There are many ways to adapt treatments in order to accommodate the sensitivities of animals. When approached without coercion and with sensitivity and flexibility, most animals, domestic and wild, will accept and appreciate a Reiki treatment. Even the most sensitive and wary animals will generally accept a distant treatment if a treatment in person is too difficult for them.

When giving a Reiki treatment, you'll typically feel deeply relaxed and may feel heat, tin-

OSCAR RELEASES HIS EMOTIONAL BURDEN

I've worked with many extraordinary animals, but some truly stand out, inspiring you with their courage and leaving an indelible imprint on your memory. One such animal was Oscar, a Russian Blue cat.

From the moment he arrived at the shelter, Oscar was severely depressed. For several weeks he rarely ate and lay with his eyes closed and his head on top of his feces in his litter box, as though making a metaphorical statement about his idea of his place in the universe. He was completely unresponsive to touch or overtures from the staff and appeared to have totally given up hope that anything could ever go well for him.

Although I didn't know the specific details of his life, I could see that he had had a particularly rough time: someone had mutilated his beautiful tail and left him with a two-inch ragged stump. The staff was very concerned about him and asked me to begin treating him.

Oscar began receiving Reiki treatments and flower essences (a vibrational remedy for emotional healing), and within days he began to improve. We first noticed these improvements when Sunny, a volunteer, was massaging him. He started to purr so quietly that we had to turn off the music in the cat area to hear him. Sunny was so touched to hear signs of life coming from him that she bent over and kissed him on top of his head. Like a person deprived of love and having almost given up on it, Oscar began to cry. For several minutes big golden tears rolled out of his eyes as he looked up at us. We praised him

gling or pulsing in your hands or elsewhere in your body as the energy flows through you. You may feel dreamy or far away at times, or may settle into a deep meditative state during a treatment. Since you're not using your own energy but the healing energy of the universe, you won't drain yourself or become sick treating others. The flow of Reiki energy through you and your animal can be dehydrating, so you should take care to stay well hydrated, whether giving or receiving treatments. Animals should have access to fresh water and may consume an increased amount of water following a treatment. Both you and your client, animal or human, can also experience increased elimination for a brief period after a Reiki treatment.

For some people and animals, a Reiki treatment will affect the emotions more than the physical being. This is because Reiki finds the issues that are most in need

for his courage in being able to open himself up and release his grief.

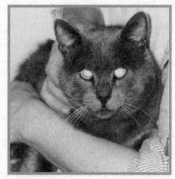

After this, he became steadily more engaged, holding our gaze and pushing against the volunteers' hands when they stroked him. He started to sit up and groom himself. Soon he was coming to the front of the cage looking for attention, batting at toys, coming out onto volunteers' laps, and looking around with interest at the other cats.

He was always exceptionally sweet and loving. When he wanted to tell someone to stop doing something, he would slowly and gently open his mouth and put it around a hand or finger so as not to upset or startle anyone. It was as though he knew from sad experience what it feels like to receive harsh feedback. After three weeks of treatment, he was alert, healthy and fully engaged in his life, and a few days later he was adopted to a good home.

I have reflected many times on the tremendous courage it took for Oscar to release his heavy emotional burden and open himself to hope and interactions with people again despite his history. But Reiki and the flower essences have the ability to reach deeply into a being to restore health and balance, and, in this case, they were aided by the love of the volunteers who took Oscar into their hearts and helped coax him back to life. —*Elizabeth*

of healing, and these may not be the issues we think need healing. Often physical problems have emotional root causes. Reiki will often go first to the deepest issues and then work "outward" through associated issues over a series of treatments.

During a treatment, Reiki is usually associated with feelings such as peace or even euphoria. However, some people and animals may experience strong emotions or cry during a treatment. This response is usually an emotional release. Reiki treatments can bring up and help release unresolved emotional issues that have been buried for many years.

Animals, like humans, can become ill when emotional matters have not been resolved and released. Reiki helps animals to let go of unresolved emotional issues and move into the present and future with a lighter heart. For this reason Reiki can be tremendously helpful for animals who have behavioral problems and/or were abused. In rare instances, animals also can weep as they release intense sadness from the past.

HEALING REACTIONS

With many energy healing systems, such as Reiki, homeopathy and acupuncture, the process of healing can involve temporary "healing reactions." A healing reaction is said to occur when the client's body temporarily produces new symptoms or intensifies old ones as it clears away infection or other injurious influences, during or after a treatment. In our experience, animals are much less prone to healing reactions than people are and exhibit them much more rarely.

THE SPIRIT OF A DOG

Sometimes the full effects of a Reiki treatment may take a few weeks to unfold. One shelter client I had was an old Akita with tumors all over her body, skin rashes, eye problems, and hip dysplasia. She had been found wandering around town when the shelter picked her up. It was clear that she'd had numerous litters of puppies. She was so sick and depressed when I arrived that she would barely wake up when people would clap their hands and call to her. I set up my chair outside the kennel, introduced myself, and began to offer the treatment.

At first, she didn't even look up, but I immediately felt Reiki flowing. I had the sense that this treatment was not about her physical body. After about five minutes, she began to have a healing reaction and scratched herself terribly. She seemed so uncomfortable! Luckily this subsided after a few minutes and she curled herself into a ball and fell asleep. After another 30 minutes of treatment, she stretched out on her side and took several huge, deep Reiki breaths.

Fifteen minutes later her mood transformed. She picked up her head, looked at me and rolled over onto her back, rolling around like a puppy, growling and grunting happily, as if she wanted me to play. Then she stood up, shook herself, looked directly into my eyes and rapidly wagged her tail! I was in shock. Then she took a huge drink of water, came back over to me and wagged her tail again, making direct eye contact. I realized that she was telling me the treatment was over, so I thanked her for being open to healing, and thanked Reiki for the amazing session.

Never would I have thought she could come around so quickly. Of course, her physical issues remained, but her spirit had begun to heal. Over the next few weeks, improvement in her physical condition followed so that she didn't even look like the same dog. Her skin cleared up, her eyes stopped running and her movement became more comfortable. Shortly thereafter, she was adopted into a wonderful home. —*Kathleen*

REIKI HEALS THE PAST

Reiki always heals the issue the animal needs most, even when this issue is not known. One of my horse clients had a very interesting reaction to a treatment I was giving for an injury to a tendon in his front leg. During the treatment, the horse had a brief but violent shaking episode, followed by a period of sleep. Near the end of the treatment, he picked up a back leg and held it in the air for some time. His person was particularly interested in this, as he had never shown that behavior before. She then shared that he had an old injury to that leg, before she knew him. Apparently he had gotten it caught in barbed wire and stood with his leg caught, and in the air, for a whole day until somebody found him. The emotional trauma of that day had stayed with the horse until, many years later, Reiki was able to help him let it go. —*Kathleen*

If a healing reaction occurs, it may initially appear that the animal's condition has worsened as a result of a Reiki treatment. For example, respiratory symptoms occasionally intensify during or directly after a treatment, and an animal that began the treatment sounding congested can briefly develop a discharge from his nose or eyes or begin coughing and sneezing. However, these intensified symptoms are brief and temporary as the body detoxifies, and they're usually accompanied by signs of recovery, such as increased energy, responsiveness and interactivity, followed by a noticeable improvement in overall health.

Healing reactions can also occur on an emotional level and, in rare instances, can result in a brief period of worsening of behavior problems before they resolve. If a healing reaction occurs, continued Reiki treatments will help it to pass as quickly as possible. Reiki can bring with it healing challenges, but in a loving, compassionate way. A healing reaction is a welcome development because it's a sign that healing is taking place.

Being a conduit for Reiki means that every time you give a Reiki treatment, you get one yourself; so it's possible, but rare, for you to have a healing reaction during or soon after a treatment. These reactions also may be on the physical or emotional level. For example, if you are coming down with a cold when giving a treatment, the symptoms may appear to worsen during the treatment but then disappear completely soon afterward.

BORIS AND NATASHA

When I came into the local shelter one day there were two new arrivals, siblings who had obviously been cared for well. The staff said that their person Amelia had brought them in earlier that day. She was going through a very stressful time in her life, and her allergy to cats had become quite aggravated, so much so that she felt she had no choice but to give them up.

Boris was a beautiful short-haired cat with distinctive black and white markings. He was energetic and impulsive, and often acted without thought for consequences. As a result, he had been hit by a car and had broken his leg a week before he came to the shelter. Still, he lay on his good side and engaged everyone with his charm. Natasha was a gorgeous long-haired white cat with brown tabby patches. She was a gentle, shy girl who huddled terrified at the back of her cage.

I gave Boris a Reiki treatment immediately to help with the healing of his leg. Later, I sent Reiki to both cats for their situation to help it resolve for the highest good for them both. The next time I stopped by the shelter they were gone, and I learned that Amelia had come and taken them home. She missed them and couldn't bear thinking of them at the shelter. She figured she would just have to find a way to deal with her allergies and high stress level.

Several days later I received a call from a young woman who had picked up my card at the shelter and wanted me to give Reiki treatments to her two cats. I had the strong intuition that the two cats were Boris and Natasha and asked her if one had a broken leg. She was quite surprised by my question but said that she wanted to help the cats let go of any negative effects from their stay at the shelter. She was again surprised when I explained that they were already familiar with Reiki.

When I arrived, Amelia explained that Boris' impulsive behavior was adding to the already high stress level she was experiencing from work. She was afraid to let him outside after his accident, and she was also concerned about whether his leg would heal well. She felt Natasha worried excessively and had been

▬ Results of a treatment

The results of a Reiki treatment can be seen in the improved health of an animal or human on any level—physical, emotional or spiritual—or on a combination of levels. Because Reiki goes to the areas that are most in need of healing, sometimes it goes beyond the being's physical or emotional body to an aspect of the being's situation. For an animal, a treatment may result in a shift in the relationship with his human

more affected by the shelter and Boris' accident than he had been. And, while Boris and Natasha had been close and affectionate all their lives, since Boris' accident, they had been in frequent conflict.

Boris immediately recognized that I was there to offer healing and licked my hands before he settled down for the treatment. He arranged himself with his head in one of my hands and his injured leg in the other. Natasha investigated what I was doing with Boris and then hid in the closet. When it was her turn she took Reiki at a distance but gradually moved closer until she was next to me with her head pressed in my hands. Boris curled up next to me while I gave her Reiki and eventually nestled under a loose shirt I was wearing.

I gave Boris and Natasha regular treatments over the next couple months. Each time I sat down and offered them Reiki, I allowed them to choose how they wanted to receive it. Each time, the one most in need of healing went first, and the other waited patiently for his or her treatment. In the beginning Boris was always first because of his broken leg, but, as the leg healed, Natasha would sometimes come forward first. Sometimes one cat would start the treatment alone and would be joined by the other toward the end of the treatment. Boris' leg healed beautifully, and he became much more grounded and less impulsive; Amelia was able to let him outside again without such a high level of worry about his safety. Amelia's allergies subsided, and Natasha bloomed into a strong, centered personality, able to hold her own in a gentle, ladylike way. Boris and Natasha became close and loving again, with each other and with Amelia. In the last year, Amelia has joined the cats for their Reiki treatments, and the whole family dozes peacefully together.

Over the past few years I have returned to work with them several times and have watched them grow into an exceptionally close and loving family. Boris now goes out through his cat door every morning around sunrise and picks flowers for Amelia from neighbors' gardens. One of her neighbors told her about watching him gently pull the blossom off a plant and carefully carry it home in his mouth. When Amelia arises, she finds blossoms artfully arranged around the house to greet her with love as she starts each new day. —*Elizabeth*

companion, within his human and animal "family unit," or in his overall situation. For instance, a Reiki treatment for an animal in a shelter environment may result in the animal being adopted, if that's what the animal needs most; or, if the animal is experiencing some difficulty in his relationship with his person, Reiki will often help to resolve the problem.

The results of a Reiki treatment are generally felt during the treatment, directly after, or over the following several days. It may become clear that there has been a physical improvement, a significant issue has shifted, an old emotional pattern has been released, or an aspect of the situation has healed. Reiki can only bring about healing and can never do harm to any being. Regular treatments facilitate the ability of the animal to deal with and eventually let go of whatever issues need healing.

While Reiki often effects dramatic changes in health, some-

DANIEL HELPS EASE THE PAIN

Eleanor called me a week after one of her cats, Rufus, had been killed by a car. She was distraught and depressed, and also worried about her other cat, Daniel, who shadowed her everywhere, had lost interest in food, and seemed depressed. She asked me to come to her home to give him a Reiki treatment.

As soon as I arrived and sat down, Daniel jumped up on my lap as though he had been expecting me. He settled under my hands immediately and fell asleep, taking an enormous amount of Reiki. Eleanor and I talked quietly during the treatment. She was experiencing serious health challenges and was disappointed that, since her diagnosis, her boyfriend of several years had been increasingly unavailable and was unable to offer her the emotional support she needed. She was lonely, sick and frightened, and felt that Daniel was trying his best to comfort her. He had taken to sleeping in the curve of her neck every night, and often seemed to be monitoring every nuance of her mood to see how she was doing.

As the treatment progressed, Reiki created a sort of cocoon around all three of us. With Eleanor's consent, I let the treatment continue beyond the scheduled hour so that she could express all the stress and sadness she was carrying with the support of Reiki. Daniel slept on peacefully. When the time came to leave, I woke him and gently put him on the bed. He licked my hand in gratitude for his treatment.

Eleanor emailed a few days later that she had a new clarity after the Reiki treatment. She told her boyfriend how she was feeling, and together they decided their relationship was no longer meeting their needs; they parted amicably. She was at peace with the decision and was working through her sadness about Rufus' death. She had several projects she was looking forward to as she recovered and was able to contemplate the future with some excitement. Daniel's spirits were higher and his appetite returned. He no longer shadowed her everywhere and took several breaks outside during the day, although he still took his job of comforting her very seriously. —*Elizabeth*

times its action is seen in other ways. For example, Reiki can ease the transition between life and death, but if it's an animal's time to leave this world, Reiki will not prevent this transition. However, Reiki frequently acts by enhancing the quality of the remaining life, by shifting the situation so that all concerned can accept the transition and let go with greater ease, and by enabling the transition to be easier and accompanied by less pain, fear and suffering.

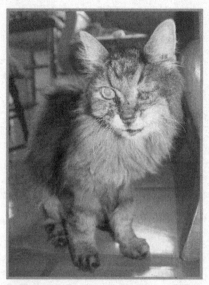

Frazier, a spry 32 years, loves hands-on Reiki treatments.

REIKI HEALS RESPIRATORY ILLNESS

For one shelter dog, Reiki healed a stubborn respiratory virus. This dog was very sick and depressed for over a month, and the drugs prescribed by the vet were having no effect. He was not expected to live. As treatment began, his eyes and nose ran and, as the Reiki treatment progressed, these symptoms worsened. He began to sneeze over and over, and huge bloody discharges flew onto the ground and all over his front paws. Then he began to cough with each inhalation, as if he couldn't take a deep breath. After this initial one-hour treatment, he was given five distant treatments in the week that followed. Within one week he was eating, playing, and able to be walked again. Within two weeks, he was adopted.

REIKI HEALS INFLAMMATION

Reiki healed a horse that was kicked in the neck. The left side of his neck had a swollen area over twelve inches long, six inches wide and two inches raised above the normal neckline. As Reiki treatment began, the horse leaned into the energy, licking and chewing in relaxation, eventually falling asleep. After 30 minutes of direct treatment, the swollen area had reduced to be about two inches long, one inch wide, and only slightly raised. With short treatments to the area twice a day, the injury was completely healed in four days.

◼ The healing timeline

In general, Reiki brings about rapid and significant health improvement. One treatment can bring about dramatic changes and sometimes be all that is needed, but more often healing is a process, and one treatment is not enough to effect complete healing. The time it takes to heal a condition can be related to the seriousness of the condition and to the length of time it has been manifest. For many conditions, a healing shift is usually apparent after one or two treatments. For acute illnesses and injuries, the sooner Reiki is received after the initial injury or onset of illness, the quicker the healing benefits will

be seen. Often, receiving a Reiki treatment soon after an injury or the onset of illness will dramatically reduce the healing time.

Chronic or long-standing conditions can require several treatments to produce significant healing results, and regular treatments for a period may be needed to continue the process. Reiki is also an excellent tool for pain management; regular treatments maintain the pain relief, and over time pain is sometimes eliminated altogether. We have seen remarkable results with conditions such as arthritic joints in both humans and animals. Additionally, when Reiki is used with other appropriate healing modalities, it often supports and enhances the effects of their combined action.

REIKI AND OTHER TREATMENTS

Reiki is a valuable component of an integrative approach to healing and health maintenance. When an animal is receiving other therapies for an illness or condition, a program of Reiki treatments can support the work of the other treatments while adding its own level of healing. For instance, when Elizabeth's dog Zoe reached the age of 16, she began to have seizures. Reiki

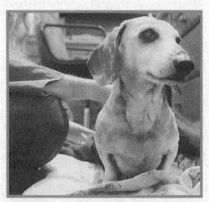

Reiki has helped Ollie, who suffers from recurrent meningitis.

REIKI EASES TAMMY'S TRANSITION

Steve and Sandra were normally a close couple who agreed about the important matters in their lives. But they were at odds about their terrier Tammy, who had a number of serious health problems and seemed to be at the end of her life. Tammy was a strong, intelligent, exceptionally personable dog who delighted in watching the animal shows on TV with Sandra and barked excitedly when her favorite shows and animals came on. She was also the mother of the couple's three other dogs. Sandra and Tammy had been best friends for nearly 15 years, and Sandra had been up every night nursing Tammy through increasingly difficult symptoms for several months.

When I first talked with Steve and Sandra, they were divided about whether it was time to assist Tammy to pass on. Sandra was exhausted, and it was painful for her to be unable to cure Tammy and to see her suffering at times. Steve felt that there was still a lot of life in Tammy and couldn't bear to end her life at what seemed to him to be a premature point. They asked me to send Reiki to Tammy to see if it would help her and to help them with their decision-making process.

I sent a series of treatments to Tammy, Steve and Sandra. Tammy's symptoms improved, and she was almost her old self for about a week. During that time Steve and Sandra got a little rest and had a chance to talk about their feelings regarding Tammy without the high level of stress that they had been experiencing. In the third week after her treatments, Tammy began to be uncomfortable again, and this time Steve and Sandra agreed that it was time to help Tammy with her transition. Tammy passed on peacefully, and Steve and Sandra were grateful for the extra time they had with her and the peace Reiki brought them in helping her to leave when the time came. —*Elizabeth*

helped with the severity of the seizures, but Elizabeth decided to try acupuncture to see if the condition could be helped further. She gave Zoe Reiki treatments before and after each acupuncture session to support its work, and after only two acupuncture treatments the seizures completely disappeared. The vet was amazed by the speed with which the results were obtained, since she had expected that more treatments would be required to get such results.

Healing from surgery often occurs more rapidly with the addition of Reiki to the treatment program. Reiki works well in conjunction with antibiotics and other medications to speed the healing of illnesses and injuries of all kinds. Reiki is a valuable component of a treatment pro-

WHERE IS CEDRIC?

Cedric, a young male cat with beautiful orange and white coloring, was brought into the shelter as a stray. His first two days at the shelter he cried and yowled constantly, clawed at his cage door, lay down in his cage and shook, fell over and pawed at the air with his legs, and even got into his water bowl and made swimming motions. He was taken to the veterinarian twice for fear this behavior was the result of seizures. No one could figure out what was going on with him, but his presence was very strongly felt in the cat area. The staff requested that I offer him a Reiki treatment. He took quite a lot of energy and became quiet and relaxed during the treatment. Afterwards he seemed a little more contained.

The next day when I stopped by the shelter I looked in Cedric's cage and saw a quiet, relaxed orange-and-white cat. I asked one of the staff, "Where is Cedric?" She laughed and said that I was one of many people who had said the same thing that morning, but that was, indeed, Cedric. Cedric stayed at the shelter for another three weeks before he found a home, but he was quiet and mellow the entire time, with no sign of his former wild behavior. —*Elizabeth*

gram for animals with cancer as well. For example, when Reiki is given before and after radiation or chemotherapy treatments, animals often experience less severe reactions and side effects. Reiki can reach deeply into the animal's being to heal emotional and spiritual imbalances that can contribute to the development and progression of cancer, as well as provide healing on the physical level. Reiki treatments can also support the animal's family as he goes through treatment for cancer.

Guidelines for Healing Animals with Reiki

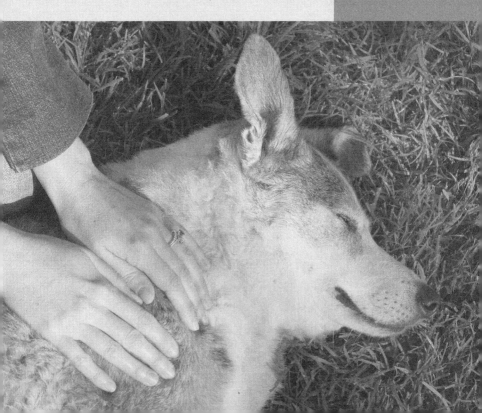

Part Two

chapter 3

Getting Ready for a Treatment

IN A SENSE, A REIKI treatment begins before you let the energy begin to flow. If you're treating an animal who is not your own, the treatment begins before you make contact with the animal or his person. By being aware of the following issues, you can make sure that by the time you begin the actual treatment, you have set the stage to provide the most effective treatment you can give.

■ Preparing yourself

It is good to be aware of your own physical and mental state when you're giving a Reiki treatment. Before giving a treatment, make sure that you have taken care of your own basic needs. For instance, try to stay well rested and make sure you are not starting a treatment on an empty stomach so that you can focus on the treatment without being distracted by your own internal state. Since the flow of Reiki through you can be dehydrating, it's a good idea to hydrate yourself before giving a treatment and to bring a bottle of water with you, if possible.

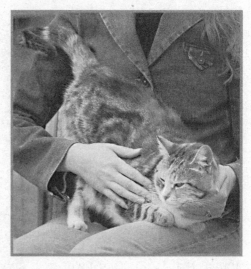

Although Reiki will work even if you're emotionally upset or physically ill, it's best to take care of yourself first before treating another, especially when working with animals. Animals will recognize and be affected by your emotional state during a treatment. If you want your animal to relax and take full advantage of the treatment without distraction from or concern about your emotions, you should calm and center yourself as much as possible before beginning a treatment. Sometimes, however, if you're upset about something and your animal is picking up on your distress, a Reiki treatment can help both of you to find a calmer, more centered state of mind and clarity about how to deal with the source of distress.

Before arriving at a treatment, take the necessary time to center yourself so that you don't bring any matters that may have been preoccupying you into the treatment, and so that you can be fully present with the animal. If you're angry, upset or even excited about something, take time to give yourself a little Reiki and to detach yourself from this emotional state. Centering yourself is especially important if you are going into a stressful environment, such as a shelter, or treating an animal who is seriously ill.

Length of treatment

It is generally best to allow at least an hour for a treatment and, if you're giving a treatment to an animal that is not your own, to plan for some additional time to discuss your impressions with the animal's person after the treatment. The length of the treatment varies with each animal, but the average treatment runs 30 to 60 minutes. Very sick animals or animals with severe emotional problems sometimes want longer treatments, or may only be able to tolerate short treatments. Allowing plenty of time for the treatment, so that you do not feel rushed, creates a calmer atmosphere, which is more conducive to a relaxed treatment for the animal.

Being comfortable

You should find as comfortable a position as possible from which to give the treatment. We have found ourselves in some very

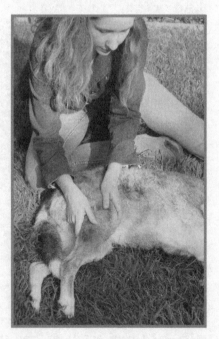

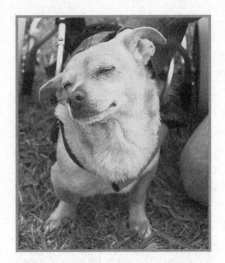

muscles to become fatigued; it's better to relax your hands on your lap if you're seated or at your sides if you're standing. Carrying a couple of stools of varying sizes in the car with you can also be useful so that you can sit at an appropriate height for the animal you're treating in any environment: a room, stall, kennel, pasture, by the side of the road or out in nature.

The treatment space

If possible, find a quiet place to give the treatment, where you will not be disturbed. A place familiar to the animal—such as a horse's stall or a small room in the animal's home—is ideal. We generally travel to the animal's environment to give a treatment, since most animals are stressed in an unfamiliar environment and are much more relaxed and at ease at home. A space where the animal can move around safely without constraints is ideal.

unusual circumstances treating animals and have learned that it's important to look after our own well-being as well as our clients' during a treatment. Try to make yourself comfortable from the outset so that you can stay focused on the treatment for its natural length of time, and so that the flow of Reiki is not impeded by your being bent into unusual positions or holding a lot of muscle tension. For example, holding your hands and/or arms up or out so that they are facing the animal can cause your

chapter 4

Giving a Treatment

EARLY IN OUR EXPERIENCE, Elizabeth's horse Annie taught us several crucial lessons about how to give Reiki to animals. Because Annie was extremely sensitive and high-strung, finding a way to approach her with Reiki was at first a daunting task. Hands-on Reiki seemed too intrusive for her, unless she was ill. During an adverse reaction to a vaccination, for instance, she leaned against Elizabeth's hands and slept for more

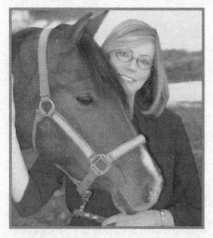

than two hours. But, more often than not, she would move away from hands-on treatments.

Once, when Kathleen offered Reiki to Annie to heal her anxiety about Elizabeth's attention to another horse, Annie walked back and forth in her stall, trying to avoid the Reiki energy. Kathleen intuitively felt that Annie was feeling coerced into receiving Reiki, so she asked Annie to take only what she was willing to receive to heal her relationship with Elizabeth. Immediately Annie stopped resisting and settled into the Reiki treatment. From that experience we realized the importance of giving an animal a choice about participating in the healing process.

By remaining flexible and open to Annie's needs, we discovered how she preferred to receive Reiki treatments. Because of Annie's conflicts about receiving hands-on Reiki, we decided to try an experiment. We stood on opposite sides of one end of her paddock, put our hands out, and let the energy flow between us, creating a "Reiki zone," and leaving the other end of the paddock a "no-Reiki zone." Annie moved back and forth from the "Reiki zone" to the "no-Reiki zone" for several minutes, but as soon as she felt that she was in control of whether she received

Reiki or not, she started positioning various parts of her body directly in the "Reiki zone." At one point, Annie started backing her hind quarters up into Kathleen's hands so enthusiastically that we were afraid she was going to sit down right on Kathleen!

Eventually, she positioned herself with her head directly between us, gradually licking and chewing (a sign of relaxation) until she nodded off. She stayed this way for nearly an hour until we ended the treatment. Since then she has spontaneously offered parts of her body for Reiki when she feels she needs it. When Annie knows she has control over the treatments, she not only accepts them but also seeks them out when she feels she needs them.

The lessons Annie taught us that day have proved to be the cornerstone of our understanding

ZOE SHOWS ME HOW TO GIVE HER REIKI

When I first learned Level 1 Reiki, I didn't have much success treating my dog Zoe. She was then about 12 and had begun to develop symptoms of kidney disease. When I placed my hands directly on her, or even six to twelve inches away, she moved away after only a minute or so, as though Reiki felt too intense for her. Eventually, I concluded that she just didn't like it and stopped offering her Reiki. Meanwhile, her kidney symptoms increased.

One day when I was standing at the kitchen sink, I suddenly felt my hands heat up and tingle. When I looked around, there was Zoe about four feet away, looking intently at me. I put aside what I was doing and stood with my hands out, Reiki pouring through them. Soon Zoe lay down on the hardwood floor, which was unusual for her since the hard surface was uncomfortable for her elderly body. But she stayed there for 30 minutes, lightly dozing.

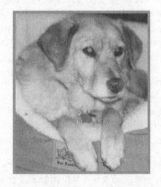

The next day she drank less, needed to go out less frequently, and looked happier and more comfortable. When we went to the vet, her lab tests showed that her urine was more concentrated. Now when she comes to me and lies down nearby with a certain look on her face, I know that she wants Reiki, generally at a distance of three to four feet. With these treatments, her kidney disease has shown very little progression. —*Elizabeth*

of how to offer Reiki to animals so that they can understand its healing potential and participate in the healing process without feeling overwhelmed or coerced. Other animals have added to the kernel of knowledge we received that day, and together, over time, our animal teachers have helped us to develop a more comprehensive understanding of how to treat animals with Reiki.

▇ Building trust

Our work with Annie and many other animals has indicated that hands-on Reiki seems to be felt much more intensely than Reiki offered from a short distance and can be experienced as invasive by animals. Some animals will refuse to participate in treatments when their only option is to have a hands-on treatment. The animals themselves have shown us that Reiki treatments are initially best given from at least a short distance. They are just as effective and often more acceptable this way, and this approach leads to more rapid establishment of trust in the healing relationship.

REIKI CALMS THE "UNCALMABLE"

Reiki has an amazing ability to bring peace to even the most stressed individual. One day at the shelter, I decided to treat a deaf Dalmatian named Spot. She was so hyperactive, constantly jumping up on me, that it took every muscle I had to keep her from escaping out of the kennel as I went inside. Interestingly, as soon as I asked her for permission to begin the Reiki treatment, she stopped whining and jumping, put her head down, stood right next to me, completely still, and wagged her tail. I had the intuition to put one hand on her heart, the other on her back between her shoulders. My hands heated up tremendously.

After several minutes, she began to scream and cry pitifully, even though she didn't move away from my hands. It was clear that she was having a healing reaction. I offered her a mental healing treatment and asked for calmness and comfort and almost immediately she quieted down. This quiet period lasted about ten more minutes and then she began to cry and move about again.

When she moved away from my hands, I felt she was ready to end the treatment. As I left, I felt thankful that at least she got a brief period of rest as a result of the treatment. I began sending regular distant treatments to her adoption situation. A few weeks later, a woman adopted Spot as a companion for another deaf Dalmatian in her household. A wonderful match! —*Kathleen*

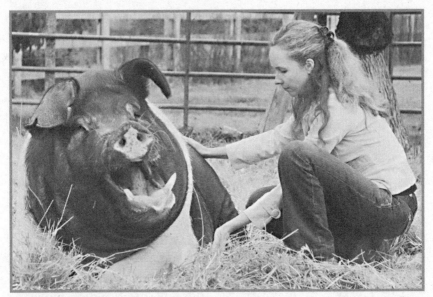
Harley yawns several times during his treatment, a sign that he's open and accepting of the healing being offered.

It's best to be patient and let go of preconceived notions of how to give the treatment, letting the animal receive the treatment on his own terms. Animals, like humans, prefer to be in control of what happens to them, especially when being introduced to a new experience. When we give an animal a treatment, our goal is to give the animal as much freedom of movement as possible and to allow him to experience and assess the healing energy in his own way, showing us how best to offer him a treatment to meet his individual needs. This approach allows animals to become acquainted with the energetic sensation of Reiki without feeling coerced. Giving animals this freedom reassures them that Reiki is beneficial and non-invasive, and builds trusting relationships with the animals. In no time at all, they usually understand the benefits Reiki offers and seek it out when they feel that they need it.

Some animals, especially our own animals who trust us already, are open to Reiki immediately. Animals with even temperaments and who have had primarily positive experiences with humans may settle down quickly and easily into receiving a treatment as well. But, like humans, animals are individuals; some are more nervous and sensitive by nature, and some have had reason to be distrustful of humans. These animals will take longer to assess the new sensation of Reiki and assure themselves that it is safe to settle into a Reiki treatment.

■ Respecting boundaries

Always be respectful of the animal's space. As you introduce yourself, stay five to ten feet away, with your arms lowered and your hands facing outward, palms forward, and allow the energy to begin to flow so that the animal can feel the energy from a comfortable distance.

Keep your hands down by your side in an offering position, since this is less threatening than holding them at shoulder level pointing toward the animal; the latter position can seem aggressive to some animals. Many animals, especially horses and dogs, will want to come up to you and smell your hands to help them assess this new sensation of energy. It's always preferable to allow the animal to come to you during a treatment, rather than approaching him; in the long run this builds trust more rapidly.

If the animal is fearful of humans, we sometimes find that visualizing ourselves keeping a

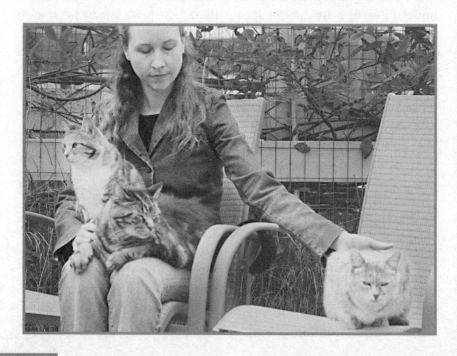

THE THREE YAWNS

Because of Reiki's powerful nature and its ability to seek out the issues that need healing, the margin of Reiki's influence often moves beyond the animal being treated. One day I was treating a horse while he was in the barn. He had been kicked by another horse, and had received terrible swollen lumps on his left shoulder and hip. The horses in the stalls on both sides of him stuck their heads out and began repeatedly yawning along with the client: all three horses, yawning over and over together! It was quite humorous to see the powerfully relaxing effect Reiki energy had on all of them. And as for my client, although the vet said the lumps wouldn't go away without being drained, they were completely gone after only two treatments. —*Kathleen*

safe distance and not attempting to make physical contact with him is helpful. From time to time during the treatment, we speak quietly and reassuringly to the animal we are treating. While we often make eye contact during the treatment, we try not to stare at the animal or force a level of eye contact that is uncomfortable for him.

■ Starting the treatment

When you're ready to start the treatment, position yourself somewhere at a short distance from the animal where he can come to your hands if he wishes. Then just rest your hands on your lap or at your sides and let the energy flow. Allow the animal to move around freely in the treatment space. Explain to the animal in a low, gentle voice that you are there to offer him Reiki energy to help him heal.

On the whole, animals become extremely relaxed, often falling asleep during a treatment. Level 2 distant Reiki is sometimes useful even in treatments given in person because it seems to be experienced as less intense and so can be good for animals who are especially sensitive to Reiki. But treating animals is usually very manageable with any level of Reiki if you allow the animal as much choice and freedom as the situation safely allows.

THE POWER OF CHOICE

As Annie first showed us, animals are more open to Reiki if they are given a choice about whether to receive it or not. When we begin a treatment, we ask the animal to take only the amount of energy with which he is comfortable.

We tell him that if he is not comfortable with the energy, he does not need to take any at all. We let him know that we will not be forcing anything upon him, including physical contact or mental connection.

In the life of most animals, humans generally determine how things will be done, on what schedule, under what circumstances, and for how long. Animals are not accustomed to being given much choice, and, when they are, they are pleasantly surprised; we often get not only the immediate attention of the animal but a deeper quality of attention from them as well. Animals become deeply engaged in the relationship with us and in the healing process.

This approach also takes into account the animal's own wisdom about what needs healing. Animals recognize the potential of Reiki healing; they will often guide us to the areas that need healing and will end the treatment when they have received enough energy to have the healing they need. Ultimately, this

LUCAS SAYS, "NOT TODAY!"

One of the horses I treat on an occasional basis, Lucas, is a beautiful chestnut Thoroughbred. He often loves hands-on Reiki, especially if he has a particular ache or pain that needs special attention. He also is a very opinionated horse and let me know on one occasion that he was not open to Reiki that day.

He had recently had dental work and, in the past, when he had Reiki after such work, he would put his mouth gently into my hands for the treatment. I approached him in his paddock, as I always do, asked permission and lowered my hands as I prepared to begin the treatment. He was relaxing on the opposite side of the paddock.

When he saw me, however, he walked briskly over and bit the air near my hands: first one palm and then the other. This behavior was new and strange to me, so it took me a minute to process the fact that he was saying, "No!" And in that moment, he actually turned around and cocked a hind leg at me, as if to say, "Is this clearer to you? Leave me alone!" I apologized to him and promptly left his paddock. He watched me go, then returned to the far corner and resumed his nap. I could tell that he was not feeling well, sore from the dental work, but obviously he just wasn't open to Reiki.

The next day was a completely different story. I returned and asked permission again. This time, he nudged me with his head, put his sore teeth into my hands, and took a deep sigh before falling asleep. —*Kathleen*

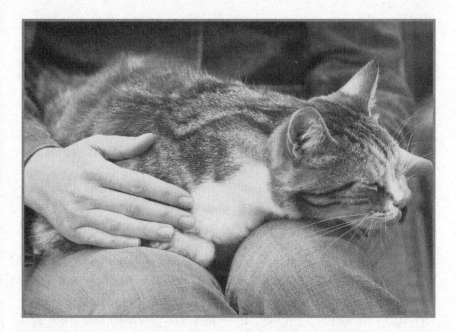

approach leads to a deeper and more intimate relationship with the animal, in which the animal can move beyond merely accepting a treatment to becoming an equal partner in a cooperative healing process.

FREEDOM OF MOVEMENT

When giving a Reiki treatment to an animal, allow him as much freedom of movement as possible within the limits of the situation. Allowing the animal to have as much control as possible over the treatment builds the animal's confidence in us and in Reiki and allows him to become an active participant in the healing process. Generally, animals will continue to move around the room (or

other enclosure) after you begin the treatment and may even move as far away as possible.

However, as they get used to the feeling of Reiki and trust that it is their choice about whether and how much to accept, animals relax and appreciate the treatment. Often, they end up positioning themselves close by or even under your hands and taking quite a lot of energy. Sometimes it will take 30 to 45 minutes for animals to settle into the first treatment, but in subsequent treatments they usually will settle into a relaxed state more quickly. There is no need to worry about whether animals are getting Reiki while they are wandering around before settling into the treatment. They will take just the amount of Reiki that they want and need during the treatment, even while moving around the enclosure.

HOW TO TELL IF AN ANIMAL DOES NOT WANT A TREATMENT

You can usually tell by the animal's body language if he does not want a treatment. If animals do not want Reiki, they will move as far away from you as they can, pace, turn away and show other signs of agitation or irritation at your presence. If they move away from you but lie down, sigh and fall asleep, they are accepting the treatment, but from a distance. By having patience, respect for the animal's point of view, and an open mind, you will find that Reiki can be adapted to be acceptable to almost every animal. In our experience, when animals are approached in this manner, they usually choose to receive the treatment.

However, if an animal does not seem to accept a treatment, then no treatment should be given. In rare instances, such as with some feral cats, especially those confined to a cage, or with animals who have been severely abused, the animal may remain too mistrustful to accept a treatment in person. Rather than force a treatment on an animal in person, you should leave and try again another day. In addition, you will sometimes find that these animals will accept a Level 2 distant treatment outside of their presence. In this case, you should offer Reiki outside of the animal's presence and leave it to the animal to decide whether and

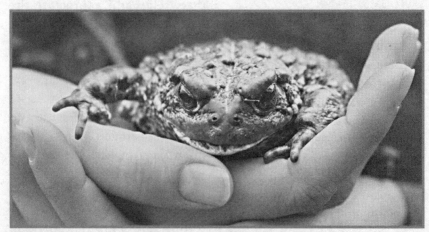

Ted the toad, usually lively, sits motionless and relaxed during his Reiki treatments.

ROSE'S REIKI MIRACLE

At the height of kitten season, when the shelter was already more than full, a very old, very sweet cat, Rose, was brought in as a stray. Rose had a number of serious health problems but was bright-eyed, seemed comfortable, and still clearly enjoyed life quite a lot. She was bedraggled and matted but appeared to be quite a lady and not a cat that had been on the streets for long. Because they were so full, with more kittens coming in every day, and because of Rose's health problems, the decision was made to euthanize her. This happens rarely at this shelter and only when circumstances become really dire. One of the volunteers asked me to send her Reiki for her transition. I did so, and also asked for the highest good for her situation, secretly hoping for a miracle.

The next day I was afraid to ask what had happened to her. It turned out that the person who was to give her the injection got sick at the last minute and had to go home. The following morning, someone who normally was not involved with the paperwork at the shelter noticed that the legally required holding period had not been met, giving Rose a several-day reprieve. Two days later a very old woman came in looking for her lost cat and, sure enough, it was Rose! The two of them went happily home together, where hopefully Rose was able to live out her days in peace. When you send Reiki you never know what the outcome will be, but sometimes it really seems that there are miracles. —*Elizabeth*

how much Reiki to receive. We discuss this further in Chapters 18 and 19.

Our goal in offering Reiki to animals is to form a trusting partnership for healing, not to get an animal to submit to a treatment or become resigned to it because he feels he has no other choice. Similarly, we do not want an animal to accept a treatment because he does not want to disappoint us. In our culture it is easy to become overly invested in whether the animal accepts a treatment and whether the animal's person sees the results she

wishes from the treatment, especially when one is just beginning to offer Reiki to animals. However, Reiki does not work like that; animals who feel pressured or coerced will not realize the full potential of a Reiki treatment and will often resist being treated.

There are many ways to give a treatment, and you can almost always find a way that will be comfortable and acceptable to your animal. In the rare instance of an animal who is unwilling to accept a treatment directly, you can send Reiki to the animal's situation, and this will provide

NANUK FINDS HER PERFECT PLACE

Nanuk was a lovely seven-month-old Malamute dog who had been turned into a local shelter as a stray. She was transferred to the local Northern breed rescue organization, where two volunteers, Laura and Adam, committed themselves to helping her to heal and find the right home. However, Nanuk had no training of any kind, was terrified of people and any indoor or enclosed space, including cars, and would immediately attack another dog. She was exceptionally intelligent and an accomplished escape artist. When she first arrived, she was severely underweight and had no familiarity with food bowls or leashes. Laura and Adam deduced from her behavior that she had lived outside and been almost totally isolated and neglected. When I met her, Laura and Adam were the only people with whom she was comfortable. They asked me to give her a series of three treatments in the hope that her chances of adoption would be increased.

During the first treatment I sat just outside Nanuk's run and offered her Reiki, asking her, as always, to take only the amount of energy with which she was comfortable. The initial thin flow of energy became a moderate one, but otherwise I could barely tell that she knew I was there. She continued her usual habit of circling rapidly around her run, jumping onto the roof of her shelter and back down repeatedly, while constantly scanning for Adam. Perhaps twice in the hour I treated her, she glanced at me for a nanosecond and sniffed almost imperceptibly at my hands once as she sped by in her circling. I was otherwise completely ignored.

Undaunted, and knowing from the flow of Reiki through me that she had accepted the treatment, I returned the following day for the second treatment. This time, when I arrived, Nanuk looked directly into my eyes for a moment and circled for five or ten minutes with less agitation. Then she lay down with her head on her paws and slept deeply for about 25 minutes. An especially loud noise woke her, and she got up and did a quick circle of her run, but then she lay down again and slept for another 15 minutes or so.

effective help for him. This is a Level 2 practice, discussed in Chapters 18 and 19.

▬ Trusting Reiki's innate wisdom

As soon as you intend for the Reiki to begin flowing (and sometimes even sooner if the need is strong), the treatment will begin. Often you will be giving a treatment for a specific health issue and so may have an intention for Reiki to heal this specific problem. However, it is important to remember that we are merely conduits for the healing energy, which has its own innate wisdom about what needs to be healed.

I sensed a strong flow of energy and was pulled deeply into the treatment until a nearby voice said, "What did you do to them? I've never seen them so quiet!" I looked up and noticed that all of the dogs in that area were asleep, despite the high noise level in the facility. After Nanuk awoke the second time, she went back to circling and searching for Adam with no further signs of interest in Reiki. The flow of energy greatly decreased, and I knew she was finished with the treatment. When I started to leave, she tried to follow me, which surprised both Laura and me.

The third treatment was uneventful. Nanuk took a moderate amount of energy, but it felt superfluous, almost as though the work that Reiki was undertaking, whatever that might be, had been accomplished in the second treatment. When I left, Nanuk made sustained eye contact, but it was not clear what the results of the treatments had been.

Two days later the rescue organization received an email from a couple who had seen Nanuk's photo and story on the Internet and had fallen in love with her. They realized that she would need a lot of love, patience and help and felt that she would teach them many things while they worked with her.

They lived in an area of California known for its year-round cool climate (perfect for a Malamute), in a beautiful home set among trees on many acres and surrounded by protected forest. The house had floor-to-ceiling windows throughout, and all of the interior materials were natural wood or stone, so that being inside was as much like being outside as possible. The couple had no children or other animals, worked at home, and immediately built her a large run so they could work on introducing her to indoor spaces as slowly as necessary. Within 20 minutes of meeting them, Nanuk bonded with the husband and stayed by his side as Laura and Adam departed.

The couple had a scare on the first full day she spent with them: Nanuk slipped her leash during a walk and ran off into the forest, but hours later she returned and walked right back up to them. After hearing the story, I felt that Reiki had truly brought the perfect home to Nanuk. —*Elizabeth*

It is best to remember that our understanding of the "big picture" is quite limited; we want to leave the door wide open for Reiki to provide the healing the animal needs most, and it may not be what we expect. For example, physical and behavioral problems are sometimes related to an emotional issue or trauma, and sometimes what an animal needs most is a shift in his situation.

One of the great things about Reiki is that we do not need to know what the source of the problem is and yet the healing will take place where it is needed most. There is no harm in forming a specific intention for a treatment, but it is Reiki's nature to provide the healing that is needed most, no matter what that may be. In our practice we simply ask for the highest good for the animal on all levels, knowing that the healing intelligence of Reiki is always superior to our limited notions of what is needed. Many times the outcome of a treatment has been much greater than anything we could have anticipated.

■ Signs of acceptance

You will be able to tell by the flow of energy through your hands, or other parts of your body, whether the animal is accepting a Reiki treatment. With Reiki, animals absorb the amount of energy they need at a rate and intensity that is comfortable for them. There are many individual variations in how animals receive Reiki. Some animals, such as those who trust people easily and those in tremendous need of healing, will take a large amount of energy as soon as the treatment begins. Animals who are more sensitive or wary will often draw only a thin flow of energy at first as they assess you and the new sensation. As they become more comfortable with Reiki, they usu-

ally draw a greater amount of energy. Some very sensitive or wary animals may draw very little or even no discernible flow of energy at first. Usually this will increase with subsequent treatments if you are patient and continue to offer Reiki as the animal tests out the new sensation.

Animals also indicate through their behavior whether they are accepting a treatment. Your animal may make sustained eye contact, push his body into your hands, lie down nearby, at your feet or against your legs, or lick and smell your hands or face if he is accepting a treatment. He may produce large sighs, deep breaths or yawns, or may doze or fall asleep. At times small animals will nestle into your hands, if they can reach them, or come directly up to the bars of the cage and lean against your hands.

Some animals will even direct your hands to the areas that need Reiki by moving their bodies around underneath your hands. Some animals show only very subtle indicators that they are accepting the Reiki energy. Sometimes nearby animals will also draw healing energy to themselves. For instance, you will sometimes look up during a treatment at a shelter and notice that, despite the high level of noise, all of the animals in nearby cages, as well as the intended recipient of the treatment, are asleep.

In most treatments, a combination of indicators will give you the best idea of how the animal is receiving the treatment; by being aware of the flow of energy and observing the animal's behavior, you can assess how comfortable and acceptable the treatment is for the animal and make adjustments, if necessary, to give him the best healing experience possible.

For instance, you may be giving a treatment to a much-loved and well-cared-for dog who was attacked by another dog and received deep lacerations on his neck and shoulder that required emergency veterinary care. He may greet you enthusiastically, tail wagging even if he cannot get up, and sigh gratefully soon after you begin the treatment. He may draw a large amount of energy to himself almost imme-

KAY AND CLARENCE

One treatment I gave to a horse taught me the value in allowing animals to choose whether or not to receive hands-on Reiki. This particular horse was a beautiful dark bay mare named Kay. She had a difficult past and needed Reiki to help her release some emotional memories. During the first treatment, I treated her from inside her stall, a few feet away. By the end of the treatment, she had pushed her chest into my hands and fell into a deep sleep, her nose lightly touching my shoulder.

However, when I approached her stall a week later for her second treatment, she moved to the far side and faced away from me, instead of greeting me as before. I decided to do the treatment sitting just outside her stall. As I began the treatment, I asked her permission and she came over to me and touched her muzzle to my hands. Then she moved back against the far wall again, lowered her head and relaxed.

At the same time, the barn cat Clarence, with whom I rarely interacted as he was so independent, suddenly appeared at my feet, meowing to come up into my lap. I placed him gently on my lap, and he immediately began purring and kneading his claws. He remained there for the entire treatment, purring loudly, while Kay periodically moved in close to touch my hands. By the end of the treatment we were all very close together, Kay standing with her nose just above Clarence's head. It was the most peaceful experience, where I felt Reiki connecting the three of us in a beautiful healing circle of energy. —*Kathleen*

THE DOG WHO NEEDED PEACE

Early on in my experiences with Reiki, one dog showed his acceptance and understanding of Reiki simply by becoming still. Tiger was an 18-month-old German shepherd who had been taken from his home due to cruelty. His collar had been left on since he was a puppy, so it had grown into his flesh, constricting his breathing. It had to be surgically removed, and his scar was just beginning to heal when I met him.

When I first approached him, he acted very much like a puppy, hyper and inattentive. I wondered if he would be open to Reiki at all. As he jumped and wiggled around me, I ran my hands gently over his body. When I put my hands over his neck injury, they heated up like fire and he went completely still, head hanging, eyes half-closed, as though someone had pushed the "pause" button on the remote. I spent the entire treatment in this one position. His complete turn-about in demeanor quite amazed me, and I was also surprised that he was open to receiving the entire treatment on his problem area. I believed at the time (and I still do) that Reiki was reaching deeply, healing not only the physical wound, but also his very heart. —*Kathleen*

diately to heal both his physical injuries and the emotional shock and hurt from the sudden attack. After 5 or 10 minutes he may yawn, put his head down and sleep soundly for the next 30 minutes while the energy flows freely to him.

A very different example would be a situation in which you are asked to give a treatment to a recent arrival at a shelter who shows many signs of past abuse and whose behavior with the staff has been unpredictable. When you sit down outside this dog's run and offer him Reiki, the flow of energy is barely discernible at first, then grows a little and drops back several times

during the first 20 minutes of the treatment.

Meanwhile the dog withdraws to the back of the run, avoiding eye contact, occasionally coming forward, walking past you and sniffing briefly at your hands without breaking stride. As long as he remains unagitated by your presence, you continue to offer him Reiki. Finally, after 35 minutes, he comes to a place about four feet away, makes the briefest possible eye contact, lies down facing you, and dozes for 15 minutes. During this time, the flow of energy increases and stays at a moderate level. In a subsequent treatment, this dog would probably take a higher amount of energy from the beginning and settle down more quickly into a relaxed state.

This example is also useful for illustrating how you would decide whether to continue the treatment in person or withdraw from the animal's presence and offer Level 2 Reiki to him at a distance (see Chapter 18). Because the dog occasionally walked past you and sniffed your hands, however subtly and briefly, and because the flow of energy picked up repeatedly, it would make sense to continue to offer Reiki quietly and patiently with the idea that the dog was testing it out and considering its potential. If, however, the dog had withdrawn to the other end of the run and his agitation had increased without any signs of interest in Reiki and with little or no discernible flow of energy, then it would have been appropriate to stop offering him Reiki in his presence and return another day, or offer Level 2 distant Reiki to him from outside his presence.

Sometimes animals will need a short period to settle down from the in-person experience (if it's not acceptable) before they will be open to a Level 2 distant treatment. In the rare instance that an animal also rejects a Level 2 distant treatment, then the animal's wishes should be respected, and no treatment should be given directly to him. You can, however, send a distant treatment to the animal's situation, and this will provide effective healing in an indirect way to the animal. In this example, it is possible that, having had his wishes respected, the dog would be receptive to a treatment in person or at a distance at a later time.

chapter 5

Hands-on Treatments

ALMOST ALL ANIMALS PREFER their first experience of Reiki energy to be at a short distance. In subsequent treatments, however, some animals will seek out and prefer a hands-on approach, moving close to or into your hands during the treatment. Additionally, an animal's preference about whether to receive hands-on Reiki or Reiki at a short distance will often shift back and forth over a course of treatments. The best approach is to tailor each treatment to the wishes of your animal during that particular treatment. This, of course, means that you need to continue to pay close attention to body language and other signs that your animal exhibits to assess his preference.

■ When to use hands-on treatment

There are several ways that your animal may indicate that he wishes to have a hands-on treatment. He may place a part of his body directly under your hands and remain there for the duration of the treatment, or he may move occasionally so that different parts of his body are

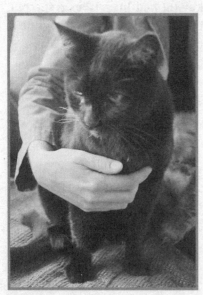

under your hands at different times during the treatment. At other times you may have a strong intuition that you should place your hands directly on your animal. In this case, if hands-on treatment is acceptable to him, your animal will show this by remaining still and relaxed under your hands and you will discern a flow of energy through you to the animal. Your animal may also seek a combination of hands-on and short distance treatment; he may move freely around the treatment area, sometimes positioning himself under or

REIKI ACCELERATES HEALING

Hamish was a dog who not only recognized Reiki but actively directed the treatments so he could heal more quickly. When I met Hamish, he was a three-year-old Lhasa Apso mix who had just had his back left leg amputated. When he first arrived at the shelter, he was so badly injured that they initially were going to put him to sleep. But, even though he was in terrible pain, he never tried to bite; his unswerving sweetness won everyone over, and they decided to try to save him.

After introducing myself and asking his permission, he turned around, facing his hind end to me. I realized he was asking for hands-on Reiki. I began the treatment by putting my hand on his left hip near the amputation stitches. |He immediately lay down, and I treated him for 45 minutes. My hands got very hot, and the hand I placed on his leg felt lots of pain and twitched constantly. Throughout the treatment, he lay completely still, sighing occasionally, awake, but completely limp and relaxed. At the end of the treatment, he turned around and gazed deeply at me for the first time. It was clearly a thank you. In subsequent treatments, as soon as he saw me he would immediately turn around, shove his left hip into my hand, and lay down for the treatment.

Soon after, I was at the shelter's party for volunteers and met a woman who began talking about Hamish, as he had become the "three-legged" mascot of the shelter, everyone's favorite. She knew nothing about my Reiki experiences with him, but she began telling me how quickly he had healed from his surgery and how everyone had been talking about the amazing recovery time. Obviously Hamish knew exactly what he was doing by backing himself right up into my Reiki hands! —*Kathleen*

near your hands and sometimes moving away during the course of a treatment. Many treatments consist of a combination of all of these scenarios.

■ Advantages of a hands-on treatment

Hands-on Reiki, when your animal prefers it, has some advantages over Reiki from a short distance in certain situations. The greatest advantage is that you will usually get more detailed information about areas of your animal's body that need healing. You may feel the flow of energy more strongly in some areas than others, indicating a higher need for healing in these areas.

This information can add to your knowledge and intuition about what needs healing and, if the animal is not your own, can be helpful to the animal's person

One of my own cats, Emma, generally prefers distant Reiki to hands-on treatments. She has always been exceptionally independent, capable, assertive and absolutely clear about what she wants. Once when her situation was quite critical, she demonstrated these qualities by taking over her Reiki treatments and directing them for her own benefit.

One day, in a fairly routine territorial dispute with a neighbor's cat, Emma got a deep puncture wound in her neck below her jaw. It became infected very quickly, and an enormous abscess formed in a place where it could easily rupture and drain back into her body, causing a potentially fatal systemic infection instead of draining safely outward and down her neck. The abscess was not responding well to antibiotics, and the usually outgoing Emma was not at all herself. She hid in the farthest corner of the farthest downstairs room under a bed, coming out only to eat, and not very often for even that.

During this period I would come down and sit in the room with her and offer Reiki to her under the bed several times a day. I would sit and talk with her, despite the fact that I couldn't even see her. One night when she seemed worse and I was really worried, she suddenly came out from under the bed very purposefully, walked over to where I was sitting, and lay down under my

in determining how to proceed with his care. This same detailed information can be obtained by using a surrogate with Level 2 distant Reiki, as detailed in Chapters 18 and 19.

Despite the more detailed information available through hands-on Reiki, the animal's comfort and preference should always be the prime consideration in whether a treatment is given hands-on or from a distance. If you disregard this consideration for the short-term benefits of hands-on Reiki, you will risk losing the long-term benefits

of establishing trust and a healing partnership with the animal.

■ Hand positions for hands-on treatment

Each treatment should be tailored to fit your individual animal's needs and preferences, which may not be typical of the majority of animals. We are including the following observations from our practice for use in customizing treatments to individual animals. Your animal's wisdom and preference should always be the primary considera-

hands. By periodically moving under my hands, she directed the treatment very methodically through several positions that together covered one whole side of her body. Then she turned over and went through exactly the same positions on the other side, finally shoving her head between my hands and keeping it there for a long time. Altogether the treatment lasted about an hour.

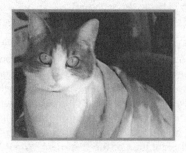

After that treatment, every time I came into the room she would come over and go through exactly the same process. It was as though she remembered the hand positions she had seen me use for humans and was adapting them as closely as she could for her own treatment!

The wound soon opened up on the outside, to our great relief, and began to drain. Soon Emma started to venture out from under the bed and into the rest of the house again. When she wanted Reiki (at least daily) she would come running up to me and meow, just like she would when she wanted to eat or go out. When she had my attention, she would run downstairs to the same chair where we started these treatments and lie down as if to say "Reiki me now!" in her typically assertive way. —*Elizabeth*

tion in the treatment, and you should feel free to depart from these suggestions when it seems to be in the interest of accommodating his needs.

Often, when an animal chooses to have a hands-on treatment, he will offer the parts of his body that need healing to your hands. If he does not indicate where he would like you to place your hands, you can start by placing your hands on a neutral area such as the shoulder. Overall it is best to pay attention to your intuition and the animal's feedback about where to focus the treatment and not to worry about the number and order of positions you use. If you find a hand position that seems comfortable for both of you, it is often best to remain in that position for the entire treatment. Once an animal has settled under your hands, changing positions will often disturb the treatment and cause the animal to become restless. Even if the animal accepts only one position for the entire treatment, Reiki will go where it needs to go to heal the animal in the ways he needs most. In our experience many treatments are best given from only one position.

THE ORPHAN

At a conference several years ago, a woman who raised orphaned kittens for a local shelter brought a litter of newborn kittens to us for a treatment because several were not thriving and their survival was in doubt. She was particularly concerned about the smallest one, who was not eating and had grown very weak. I treated the little mass of kittens in a towel on my lap with my hands cupped several inches from them. The weakest kitten inched its way over to one of my hands and fitted itself into the curve of my hand, staying there for the duration of the treatment. When I called the woman at the end of the week to see how the kittens were doing, she reported that all were eating well, gaining weight, and were expected to survive. —*Elizabeth*

Human treatments traditionally begin with hand positions on the head and move downward over the torso, but we have found that for animals, hand positions on their head are often not comfortable. Some animals will accept your hands on their head at the end of the treatment after they have become accustomed to the Reiki energy, but it is often better to place your hands on an animal's head only when he pushes his head into your hands or indicates in another way that this is what he wants. Animals will sometimes lie down a foot or two away with their head near your hands when they want Reiki for their head, and this seems to be more comfortable to them. We have found a favorite hand position for many animals is placing one hand on the animal's chest and the other on the middle of the back at the shoulders. This is also a good position for focusing on the heart, which often seems to be the center of emotional healing.

Sometimes it is possible to proceed through a sequence of hand positions similar to human treatments; however, often the area in particular need of healing, such as arthritic hips, areas of old fractures, etc., will be sensitive, and the sensation of Reiki directly on the area will be too intense for the animal. This seems to be particularly true of injured bones and joints. In this case, placing your hands on a major joint above the affected area will often be acceptable and even comforting for the animal.

For example, placing the hands on or slightly above their

shoulders is usually acceptable for dogs with hip dysplasia (an inherited condition in which the hip joint does not fit together well). Placing the hands on or near the spine over the affected leg is usually acceptable for horses with hind-leg arthritis. In contrast, an animal will often accept your hands directly over a muscle, organ or tissue in need of healing, and the sensation of Reiki in this case often appears to be soothing.

A very sick animal, or one who is in severe pain, may be willing to accept your hands only at some distance from the area that is painful or uncomfortable. For instance, a horse with colic (discomfort in the digestive tract)

GRANT SEES HIS WAY IN LIFE

Grant was a large, handsome, 16-month-old golden Labrador. He had begun life with the idea that he would become a guide dog for the blind, but at about a year of age it was decided that he was not well-suited to that kind of life. When I met him, Grant was highly anxious, hyper-vigilant and constantly in motion. He had a short attention span and had not outgrown the need to mouth everything, including the hands and arms of the people around him. He was easily excited and, when excited, would sometimes mouth too hard and hurt someone. He was not in any way aggressive but in his excitement sometimes got carried away.

His trainer Maddie was devoted to him and committed to finding the right home or situation for him. She chose him for a demonstration treatment because he had been so difficult to help and had shown less progress than expected up to that point. We found a quiet room and put our hands out and let the energy flow, asking Grant to take only the energy he wanted.

At first Grant moved around the room with his customary anxiety and agitation; he would come back to us and settle briefly near our hands and then go off exploring the room and looking for anything that might serve as a play toy. After 10 to 15 minutes, he came over and lay down at our feet with his head directly under my hands. Soon he sighed deeply and went to sleep. He remained there for the rest of the treatment, about another 30 minutes. Then he got up, gazed into my eyes, licked my hands gently, and re-embarked on his exploration of the room, with considerably less anxiety and agitation.

Maddie gave him regular Reiki treatments for several months along with the other training techniques that she used, and when I next saw him, he was a changed dog: calm, quiet and attentive. —*Elizabeth*

may not want your hands on her abdomen but may accept and appreciate your hands on her neck or shoulder. An animal with a severe laceration on his front leg may not want your hands near the injury but will relax and go to sleep if your hands are placed on his hip.

Flexibility is important in treating animals; you should not be afraid to experiment to see what works best for each animal and each treatment. Sometimes, your animal will want or accept hands-on Reiki, but feel uncomfortable with both of your hands, still and unmoving, on him. If this seems to be the case, stroking the animal with one hand while leaving the other one in one place to give the treatment is often much more acceptable. Alternatively, keeping your palms on your animal and lightly scratching, stroking or rubbing him with your fingers will often be acceptable. Sometimes your

TESS TELLS ME WHAT HURTS

One of my clients was a beautiful white pony named Tess. As I began the treatment, I introduced myself to Tess and explained that I would be offering her Reiki, with her permission. I stood several feet away since this was her first treatment and I didn't want to startle her with the new sensation of the energy. After a few minutes, she approached my hands and began sniffing them. It was clear that she felt the energy and was very curious about it.

Because she remained standing close to me, I tried hands-on positions in various parts of her body to see if I could feel any energetic changes in my hands that might correspond with her lameness problem. As I moved my hands to her shoulder, I told her that I was listening if there was anything she wanted to share with me about her soreness. She became very still as I moved my hands from her shoulder, down her back to her hind end and legs. Then I moved to her front right knee. My hands heated up as I settled in this position. Simultaneously, Tess lifted her right leg in the air and held it there for a moment. When she returned her hoof to the ground, she pushed her muzzle against her knee, then against my hands, and then against her knee again. Reiki had found the problem area.

I spent about 20 minutes in this one position, and her head lowered almost to the ground and she fell asleep. When I moved to the other side, she reacted some to the knee area, but less strongly. Finally, she roused from her relaxed state and moved away from my hands, ending the treatment. With some stall rest and continued Reiki treatments, she recovered quickly. —*Kathleen*

SENEDAD SEEKS REIKI

One of my own horses, a beautiful Arabian mare named Senedad, seeks out Reiki from me when she feels she needs it. When I first became her person, I learned that she had a number of dental problems, which I took care of as soon as possible. The dentist had to pull two of her teeth and do some other work. Unfortunately, Senedad was even more uncomfortable for a short while after the dental work than she had been before.

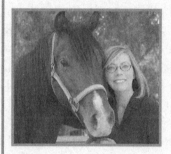

Reiki seemed to be like a life raft for her through this time, giving her comfort and healing for body and soul. During this period of discomfort she sought out Reiki often. She would rest her head against my chest while I put my hands on her jaw, or would lie in her stall with her head in my lap and her jaw in my hands for as long as I could give her Reiki. We were both glad to have Reiki to get her through this difficult time. —*Elizabeth*

animal will prefer your hands to be five or ten inches away from his body for some or all of a treatment.

■ When to use Reiki from a short distance

Animals may come to your hands and move away during a treat-ment. If your animal moves away, you can find a place several feet away in the treatment area to stand or sit and offer Reiki. Your animal may come back to your hands, stay at a distance, or come and go throughout the treatment. He will receive the healing he needs whether he is directly under your hands or at a short distance.

chapter 6

Insights during Treatments

IN THE COURSE OF GIVING treatments to animals, you may receive insights about what needs healing, and these insights can take different forms. They may come in the form of physical sensations felt during the treatment or in the form of emotional information communicated from the animal during the treatment. The different forms of insights are just different ways of guiding you to what needs healing for the animal. Often you do not need to do anything with the information you receive because the wisdom of Reiki will guide the healing to the matters of greatest need. Sometimes, however, the insights will indicate some action that will help to move the healing more rapidly or will broaden the scope of healing.

■■■ The meaning of physical sensations

As described in the previous chapter, when you give a Reiki treatment, hands-on or distantly with a surrogate (see Chapter 19), you may receive detailed information about the parts of the body you are treat-

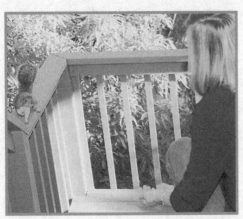

ing. Specifically, you may become aware of an increased flow of energy or physical sensations (such as heat, pulsing or tingling) in your hands, arms or other parts of your body. This increased flow generally means that the area under your hands has a higher need for healing. A sensation of cold in a part of the body also may mean that the area has a greater need for healing. Occasionally, you may temporarily feel an ache or pain in your hand, arm

MAY AND JACK

May and Jack were three-year-old sister and brother cats. They had been left alone in an apartment for two weeks before a neighbor realized she had not seen anyone come and go and called the local animal shelter. They had had water from the toilet but no food and were very thin. Both May and Jack were frightened of people and cringed when anyone came near, but May was especially scared; Jack would curl his body around her as they lay at the back of the cage, as though trying to protect her from danger as best he could.

I gave them several Reiki treatments from a short distance. Each time the same image of a sunny window in a corner with a window seat covered in soft cushions and sunlight on the adjoining wall would form in my mind. I always seemed to see it from across the room, in a doorway. The image was accompanied by a peaceful feeling and then a sense of longing. Each time I offered them Reiki for individual healing, I would also send Reiki to their situation in the hope that the right home would come to them.

After a couple of weeks, a man came into the shelter looking for his two cats. He had left them with someone he thought was trustworthy while he was out of town and was horrified when he could find neither caretaker nor cats on his return. He, May and Jack were overjoyed to see each other, and, as they departed, I found myself hoping that they were going home to the soft, sunny window seat in the corner. —*Elizabeth*

or another area of your body during a treatment. This sensation, like cold or heat, usually means that the area you are treating on the animal at that time has a higher need for healing. This pain is not your own pain and will disappear quickly when the treatment ends.

When giving hands-on treatments, try to stay in the position where you feel the increased sensation until it begins to subside before moving on to another position. If you move through a series of positions, you may notice that some areas show a higher need for healing than others. However, please keep in mind that a healthy being with a high affinity for Reiki can also absorb a large amount of energy, so the absorption of a great deal of energy does not necessarily mean that there is a critical illness or injury. You should always weigh the physical information you receive in light of other factors, such as the animal's appearance and behavior, your own intuitive sense of the situation, and any information you have from the animal's person, if the animal is not your own companion.

Similarly, when you are giving a treatment from a short distance, you may feel the energy through your hands or other parts of your body increase and decrease over the course of a treatment. When working with an animal who has a high need for healing, initially the flow of energy may be quite strong. This is especially true if the animal has had mainly positive experiences with humans, is relatively trusting of them, and is open immediately to the new sensations of Reiki energy. Or the energy may start off at a low level as the animal tests out and becomes acquainted with the energy. It generally becomes stronger later in the treatment as the animal becomes comfortable, settles into the treatment, and begins to absorb the energy more confidently. Sometimes a high degree of comfort with the energy does not occur until the subsequent treatment. In a treatment from a short distance, you can sometimes get a level of detailed information similar to that available through a hands-on treatment by visualizing the energy going to a series of positions for different areas of the animal's body, as though you were giving a hands-on treatment.

A STORM OF EMOTIONS

When I met Franny, she had been at the shelter for several weeks. She was a young cat who had probably lived outside for most of her life, and had been brought in as a stray. When she arrived at the shelter, she was in an advanced stage of pregnancy. Because it was "kitten season" and the shelter was often short on space, Franny's kittens were aborted.

Although she was shy and wary when she arrived at the shelter, she could be handled and held by the more experienced volunteers. After she lost her kittens, no one could touch Franny. She was deeply depressed, and rarely moved or ate. She wanted nothing to do with people. The staff asked me to treat her for her profound depression.

I sat by Franny's cage, talked to her quietly and offered her Reiki, asking her to take only the amount of energy she wanted. At first I thought she would refuse the treatment because there was such a thin, weak flow of Reiki. Eventually, however, she drew in an enormous amount of energy. Franny stayed on my mind all week, and I felt her loss strongly.

◼ Emotional information

While giving a treatment, you may also get visual images, thoughts or feelings about matters pertaining to the animal, including previous losses or traumatic experiences. Often these images, thoughts or feelings are related to what the animal needs in order to heal. Sometimes you may even feel what the animal is feeling or what he once felt in the past. These experiences can sometimes be very strong and can be disconcerting at first. It can be helpful to remember that the feelings do not actually belong to you; they are just information from the animal, and

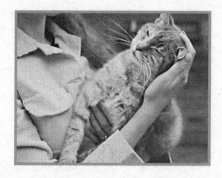

they will go away when the treatment ends.

One of the strongest emotions Kathleen received during a treatment came from a dog with aggression problems. She sat on the ground next to him, introduced herself and began to offer Reiki. He leaned against Kathleen and sighed. After about 20 minutes, for a brief moment Kath-

---

A week later, as I put my hands out and let the energy flow, I was nearly swept away by a storm of emotions. I could sense—almost feel—a gale-force wind blowing and see it bending palm trees almost to the ground. I could see flickers of light all around, which put me in mind of an electrical storm. I knew this was coming from Franny and took it as a good sign that she would entrust me with this emotional storm. I stayed with the storm and envisioned it gradually becoming a medium hurricane, then a strong storm, then a very windy day, then a breezy day, and finally a calm day at the beach, with the waves lapping the shore and a warm sun beating down. When I got to the last image, I felt Franny had vented and released a great deal of emotion. I apologized to her from the bottom of my heart on behalf of my species for what had happened to her kittens.

At the end of the treatment I felt there was reason for hope and told the staff. They tried to take Franny out of her cage and were amazed when she came out easily, purred, rolled over on her back, allowed herself to be brushed for the first time, and was generally very sweet. In subsequent treatments, I received images of sparking, commotion and wind for a minute or so but never anything like the sustained intensity of the "storm." —*Elizabeth*

THE CAT WHO WAS AFRAID OF DOGS

One day at the local shelter I was led to a very agitated, young black-and-white cat. The staff person, Katie, was concerned that no one would want to adopt him because he was so nervous he couldn't be held. She wondered if Reiki could do anything for him.

I stood by his cage and offered him Reiki. I soon got a picture of a dog on a leash coming through the cat building door, combined with the words "Danger!" and "Dog!" I noticed as well that the cat kept straining and trying to look into the back room of the cat area in a nervous, fearful way. I asked Katie if dogs ever came into the cat building. She said dogs were never allowed, but my feelings persisted.

When Katie asked if there was anything she could do for the cat, I suggested that she tell him as often as possible that it was safe there and that dogs never came in. I said it might also be helpful to take him into the back room and let him see what was there. She proceeded to do this, telling him all the while that he was safe and dogs were never allowed in the cat area. She was surprised when he settled down in her arms, purring, and sat quietly when he was returned to his cage.

Later that day I got a phone message from Katie saying that the cat was still quiet and affectionate. She had just learned that a new volunteer, unaware of the rules, had indeed taken a dog into the cat building the day before, just after the cat had arrived. After his treatment and tour of the back room, the cat remained quiet, affectionate and easy to handle, and easily found a new home within a few days. —*Elizabeth*

leen's head spun and it felt as if her heart was breaking. She thanked and acknowledged the dog for sharing this with her. He immediately got up and moved far away, facing the other direction. He was finished with the treatment.

Kathleen told his people what she had experienced. They proceeded to tell her how they adopted him. They found him in the street with a head injury caused by some terrible abuse. Although he appeared recovered, he had a split personality, sometimes shifting from loving and gentle to vicious for no reason. After Kathleen heard their story, it was clear to her that the memory of this injury was what she had experienced while treating the dog.

After the treatment, Kathleen sent several distant treatments to help the healing process. His people were amazed at the immediate improvement in his behavior after the Reiki treatments. He was a changed dog! In the weeks that followed, he needed daily Reiki treatments to prevent his aggression from coming back.

It can be difficult, especially at first, to distinguish communications from the animal from your own hopes, preconceptions and projections. As healers, we all need to do our best to be aware of our own feelings and issues so that they do not influence the treatments we give to animals, nor cloud the information we might receive from them. Because of their sensitive natures,

animals can feel pressured, distracted and overwhelmed by our emotional states. Such feelings might cause them to reject the Reiki treatment we offer. It is also possible that we project our own emotional challenges and issues onto our animal, causing a misunderstanding of what's really going on with them.

This is one of the reasons self-treatment and receiving treatments from others are so important in our growth and development as Reiki healers. Our own treatments help us heal more deeply and become as clear and open as possible as conduits for Reiki energy. As we heal our-

THE WISDOM OF BOSLEY

Bosley was a very wise-looking white cat in New York to whom I sent distant treatments. She had an advanced cancer in her lower jaw and her devoted person Mark wanted to do everything he could to help her to be as comfortable as possible through the last period of her life.

The first Reiki treatment helped Bosley a lot; Mark reported that she became much more her old self afterwards and seemed to be more comfortable. When she became uncomfortable again, he asked me to send another treatment. This time, when I was deep in a meditative state, I suddenly became very nauseated. I had an accompanying intuition that this was caused by medication that she was on. I thanked Bosley for the information.

When I spoke with Mark, it turned out that she had vomited several times in the last week and that she was taking quite a few conventional and alternative medications. Mark consulted with her veterinarian and her homeopath, and they cut out all medications except those to help Bosley be comfortable. The next time I sent a treatment to her, she seemed peaceful and comfortable, and Mark reported that she was more active and enjoying life more. —*Elizabeth*

selves, the energy can flow through us as strongly and purely as possible for the greatest benefit to animals.

Intuition and communication

Often, over time as you use Reiki with your animals, your intuition deepens, sometimes dramatically, and you can become able to receive more information from your animal, especially about

healing. When your animal shares information about his state of mind or previous difficulties in life, it is a sign of trust and a great honor for you to be entrusted with this knowledge. Being able to share this information with you often enables your animal to begin to release these feelings and memories, accelerating mental and emotional healing and helping him to move on in his life.

A DOE AT THE DOOR

The first thing that attracted me about our house was that it backed up to the greenbelt that ran down from the hills toward the San Francisco Bay. Behind our house is a large undeveloped parcel that is a haven for a wide variety of wildlife. I often saw deer passing through or stopping and resting there. I recognized that their lives in our suburban neighborhood were tough, so when I saw them outside I sent Reiki to them from the window, for a few minutes whenever I could.

Early one morning, after I had been doing this for about a year, my husband burst into the bedroom, astonished and upset. Each time he tried to take our dog Zoe out for a walk, he was charged by a doe standing just outside our front door. Unbelieving, I went to the front window and looked out. Indeed, there was a very agitated-looking doe there, eyes wide, nostrils flaring.

As I looked at her, the word "baby" formed in my mind. At first I thought she was pregnant and about to give birth. I told her it was all right, that no one would hurt or disturb her, and she was safe there. As I spoke, she visibly relaxed and, as she did so, a very blurry image of a small, curled being came into my mind. I looked around our courtyard and saw a fawn, still curled and covered with amniotic fluid, lying in the wood chips a short distance away. We left the doe and her fawn undisturbed, and my husband and the dog left by the back door. I realized that these ideas and images had come from the doe, and I was incredibly excited by this brief exchange with such a glorious creature. Later that day I sent Reiki to the doe and her fawn for their protection and general well-being.

In addition, when your animal shares this type of information, it shows that you are doing an excellent job of establishing a healing partnership with him. This is one of the main reasons we encourage people to take great care in establishing a healing relationship with their animal. By giving your animal as much choice and freedom of movement as possible and by listening to and respecting his wishes and concerns, you communicate to him that you are someone who can hear and understand his problems on a level that many others have not yet tuned into. Your animal begins to understand that you are able to offer a kind of help that has not been available to him before. He further understands that he can obtain this help without giving up his autonomy or undergoing stress or discomfort. He learns that he can be an equal partner in his own healing

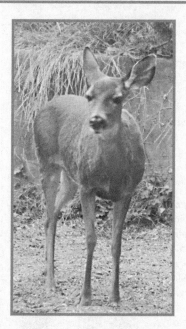

The next morning I ventured outside to see if we could have another encounter. I roamed the area near my house, sometimes calling out softly to her, sometimes calling to her internally. After a while I gave up and, as I turned abruptly back onto the sidewalk, I almost knocked the doe over. She had heard me and was standing right behind me! We gave each other a tremendous scare, and she leaped to the other side of the street. We stood looking at each other for a long time. No words or images passed between us, but a gentle, vibrant energy and feelings of love connected us. I felt that both of us were re-evaluating our ideas about relationships between our species, and a bond was being forged between us.

This encounter was the first time I clearly recognized that I was communicating with animals, and I went on to fully develop this ability. To this day I feel that the doe chose our courtyard to deliver her fawn because of the healing energy of Reiki she had felt coming from our house on so many occasions. In addition, I credit Reiki with helping me to learn how to rest in a calm inner state and tune in to the "language of energy" so that animal communication could begin to take place. —*Elizabeth*

and can guide you in helping him to have the healing he needs without stress. One of the ways he may try to guide you is by sending emotional information. Other ways include physical sensations and placing the parts of his body in need of healing directly into or near your hands.

For many people, realizing that they are receiving a deeper level of communication from their animals fulfills a long-time dream and provides them with further clarification as to why the care they have taken in establishing a healing relationship with their animal has been worthwhile. It often opens a new level of understanding and intimacy in their relationship with their animals. These expanded possibilities are a direct result of Reiki's ability to enhance individual intuitive gifts and our own efforts in listening to them and allowing them freedom of choice.

A RESTFUL NIGHT'S SLEEP

One of my cats, Mu Shu, came to me soon after she was separated from her kittens. Her person had moved out of state and had left her with a local vet, who had separated them and agreed to find homes for them all. Mu Shu settled in quickly, a much-loved addition to our household. She never slept for very long, however, especially at night. She would spend much of the night wandering from room to room. When I learned Reiki, Mu Shu became "a Reiki sponge": Every night I would find her waiting for me, and she would soak up Reiki for as long as I was able to give it to her.

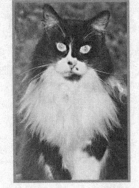

When I was deep in a "Reiki state" during one of these sessions, I had the sudden strong conviction that Mu Shu was still worried about her kittens. I called the vet's office and they assured me that they always found homes for the animals they took on. During my next Reiki session with Mu Shu I told her that I learned that her kittens were safe and in good homes, so she didn't need to worry about them anymore.

I didn't think much more about this until a couple of nights later, when I realized that Mu Shu no longer wandered and had been sleeping peacefully through the night ever since I talked with her about her kittens. To this day she sleeps soundly all night long, and I believe it's because her mind is finally at rest about her kittens. —*Elizabeth*

THE GOOD CHICKEN

One day at the shelter, I was drawn to a big, white chicken who was huddled in the back of the cage. One of the staff explained that he had been adopted as a chick, but when he grew up to be a rooster instead of a hen, his person could no longer keep him. It was clear that the bird was emotionally distressed, so I offered him a mental healing. I introduced myself and let him know that I was here to help him heal and listen if there was anything he wanted to share with me. To be honest, I didn't expect that chickens thought about many things, except perhaps seeds.

As I felt the energy flow increase, I suddenly had a clear picture of this chicken's emotional state. He was very distressed that he was at the shelter because he believed that he had been a very good chicken and couldn't understand why his person had sent him away. I mentally told him that he was brought here because that just wasn't the right home for him, but that he was a very good chicken in every way, and in fact was very beautiful. Amazingly, as soon as I told him this, he got up from the corner of the cage, came right up to the front of the cage and began to cluck at me and happily strut back and forth. In this case, offering a mental healing treatment not only relieved the chicken, but also taught me a valuable lesson in not underestimating the depth of any animal's understanding. —*Kathleen*

It is not necessary to receive communications from our animals in order to establish a strong healing relationship with them. Not every Reiki healer will receive communications from her animal. Some people appear to have more of a natural affinity for receiving communications, and Reiki will generally accelerate the development of this ability as it deepens the healer's intuition.

However, Reiki heals very effectively regardless of whether you receive information from your animal, and people who do not receive such information are able to heal just as effectively as those who do receive it. In using Reiki with animals, your particular areas of strength are enhanced in ways that will show you new possibilities with animals as well.

A Reiki treatment provides an extended period of quiet time for you and your animal to spend together. It can be experienced by your animal as a time when he can share some of his innermost concerns by sending you information about his physical and emotional well-being through physical sensations or emotional insights. After your animal has

SMOKEY LEARNS TO TRUST

Smokey was a middle-aged, gray, feral cat who had been brought to the shelter three months earlier by a woman who had been feeding him for a year. She was moving and feared there would be no one to feed Smokey. Smokey hated the shelter, did not want to be handled, and tried to escape several times. He was very wary of people and often bit volunteers who tried to socialize him.

When I met him, the staff was very concerned because after three months in the shelter he sat hunched in one corner, never moving and severely depressed. He started at every noise and movement, and, although he could be taken out of his cage by a few of the most experienced volunteers, he would lunge for and bite people's faces as soon as they came into view.

I worked with Smokey for several weeks, sitting on a chair outside his cage, my hands in my lap. In the first treatment, Smokey accepted Reiki readily and allowed himself to doze lightly, but each time there was a noise, or even the slightest movement of my hands, he would jolt himself awake.

During the second treatment, while I was deep in the meditative state often induced by giving Reiki, I received a strong impression of a blow to the head. I also felt certain that Smokey was very sensitive to light and this was related to the blow. I thanked Smokey for telling me this and told him how sorry I was that this had happened to him and how courageous he was in reaching out to me.

I told the staff my intuition about Smokey and suggested they try working with him with the light off, in just the dim light from the adjacent room. When they tried this, Smokey came out readily and no longer lunged toward faces. There were no more biting incidents. He was still a cat to be handled only by the most experienced volunteers, but with them, he was an angel. He began to move around his cage, come to the front, and roll over on his back playfully and touch people gently with his front paws.

informed you about his health and state of mind, he can often show an immediate and marked improvement in any symptoms he has been exhibiting. For example, an animal who has refused food may suddenly go find his bowl and begin to eat.

Animals in your household who normally do not get along may make peaceful contact during or after a treatment. Or, if your animal is fearful, the treatment may begin with him hiding out of sight, and during the course of the treatment you may see him

During his sixth Reiki treatment, for the first time he allowed himself to go deeply into a relaxed state and sleep, oblivious to the noises and movements around him. The next time I came, he was sound asleep, so much so that the volunteers had to tap on the cage bars and raise their voices to get his attention. He opened his eyes briefly, stretched toward me, and went back to sleep.

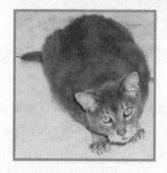

Smokey had recurring dental problems, and his next trip to the vet determined that he was almost blind and that his vision and dental problems had been caused by a blow to the head. There was a large area of calcification on the side of his jaw, where the vet felt the blow had landed.

When the shelter learned that Smokey was nearly blind, they began to understand his point of view. As a feral cat who had been seriously injured, he was understandably wary of people. This wariness was compounded by his limited vision, which left him feeling vulnerable at all times. When people took him out of his cage onto their laps and he looked up at their faces, he was blinded by the strong fluorescent light just over their heads in the small room. Frightened because he couldn't see, he reacted defensively by attacking in the direction of the light.

Now there was an outpouring of love and sympathy toward Smokey. Basking in this love and feeling understood, Smokey relaxed and became affectionate with his favorite people. I became unusually attached to Smokey and let him lick baby food off my fingers before or after a treatment, something I never do, but Smokey was extra special. Smokey loved his Reiki, however, and generally chose to have Reiki first and the baby food after his treatment. For a cat who was very possessive of his food and had difficulty allowing people to remove and refill his food dish, this was a high compliment indeed! —*Elizabeth*

venture bravely out into view. Issues that have been present for a long time may require repeated Reiki treatments for the full healing effects to be seen or for the improvements to become steady and permanent. Over time as you spend intimate Reiki time with your animal, allowing him to share his concerns with you through physical and emotional insights, you will be able to add new and important dimensions to your understanding of him, deepening your communication and bond with one another.

chapter 7

Ending the Treatment

■ How to tell when a treatment is coming to an end

IDEALLY, YOU WILL ALLOW yourself enough time when giving a treatment so that the animal clearly becomes relaxed and at peace. The animal may give several long sighs (or "Reiki breaths," as we call them) and will generally become deeply relaxed or fall asleep. Once this level of connection with Reiki has occurred, the deepest work of the treatment often takes place.

For this reason, at this point in the treatment you should not move your hands if you are giving hands-on Reiki. If you are offering Reiki from a short distance, you can just sit quietly and allow the Reiki to flow. Often when your animal comes out of this state of deep relaxation, he will have received the healing that he needs and will indicate that he is ready to end the treatment.

Since animals cannot tell us in words when they are finished with the treatment, we have to learn to read their body language and facial expressions to be as sensitive to their wishes as possible. Once you feel a dissipation of the energy flow, you should give the animal a few minutes to show signs that he is also finished with the treatment. The animal will often indicate this by waking up, moving away, becoming occupied with something else, or by offering you a gesture of thank you. An animal can show thanks in many ways, such as licking your hands or face, gazing deeply into your eyes, putting a paw on your arm or leg, touching his head to your hands or chest, or making happy, satisfied sounds, such as nickering, purring, grunting or squeaking.

Some animals do not reach a state of deep relaxation, especially in the first treatment, but they will receive the healing they need in the treatment all the same. In subsequent treatments, when they have become familiar with Reiki, they will usually become more deeply relaxed.

When an animal does not become deeply relaxed, there are other ways in which you can tell that the treatment is ending. If you are giving Reiki from a short distance, you may feel a marked decrease or cessation of the flow of energy in your hands or other parts of your body. If you are giving a hands-on treatment, especially from one hand position only, you will feel a similar decrease in the flow of energy. If you have given a series of hand positions, you will feel the energy decrease in the last position. If you are not yet able to feel the flow of energy, you can just go by the clock and end the treatment after about 45 minutes to an hour.

Another way you can tell that the treatment is coming to an end is by your own state of awareness as well as changes in the flow of energy. When you feel yourself come out of a deep meditative state, or when your attention begins to wander to other matters unrelated to the treatment, these are often signs that the healing work of the treatment is coming to an end.

INDICATORS THAT AN ANIMAL IS READY TO END THE TREATMENT

If your animal indicates that he has had enough before you feel a reduction in the flow of energy, you should listen to the animal and end the treatment. The ani-

EMMA'S LESSON

Sometimes my cat Emma participates in my Reiki classes, helping me teach by allowing students to give her Reiki treatments. On one particular day she did not show up to volunteer for this job. Toward the end of the class, she stretched out on the deck outside the class. I went out with a student to see if Emma would let her give her a treatment, but as we went out, Emma went up the stairs to the upper deck. When we followed, she reluctantly let the student offer her Reiki.

After a few minutes she got up and licked the student's hands, walked away and lay down a foot or so away. The student moved over, put her hands on her and continued to send Reiki to her. Emma bit her softly, without breaking the skin, but drawing a clear boundary for us when we had ignored the other, more polite signals she had given us. The student understood immediately, was not upset, and felt that it was a good lesson for her. It was a useful reminder for me as well not to take advantage of Emma's occasional generosity in helping to teach a class. —*Elizabeth*

THE DOG WHO THANKED REIKI

Malty was an extremely timid and nervous five-year-old stray Maltese, described by employees at the shelter as "in really bad shape." His tongue hung out all the time and he was so thin you could feel every bone. He wore a little green sweater to keep warm. Once I took him into a quiet room for his treatment, he really seemed to want Reiki. He stood absolutely still, except for his constant shaking, leaned against me and rested his tongue and head on one of my hands, while I put the other hand on his back near his tail.

I felt a tremendous amount of Reiki flowing through my hands despite his small physical size. By the end of the hour, he actually stopped shaking and his breath got very deep, with periodic sighs. He also began to expel some gas (another common effect of a Reiki treatment). At the end of the treatment, he looked up at me quite seriously and, while holding my gaze, put one paw on my leg as if to say, "Thanks!" —*Kathleen*

mal's wisdom about what he needs is quite accurate and, in any event, you will encourage the growth of trust in the relationship for future treatments by listening to the animal's wishes. In rare cases, an animal may give a warning or actual bite if you do not end the treatment after the animal has indicated he has had enough. Sometimes your animal will continue to sleep after you feel the energy dissipate. In this case, just leave quietly, allowing the animal to continue sleeping until he awakes naturally.

EXAMPLE OF AN END TO A TYPICAL TREATMENT

Say you are giving a Reiki treatment to a cat. For the first 30 minutes, the cat gets up and lies down repeatedly, plays with a toy, and walks around the space, from time to time coming back to or near your hands. Finally, after half an hour, the cat lies down directly under your hands, sighs twice and falls asleep. He remains motionless and completely at peace for another half an hour. Then, suddenly, he wakes up, licks your hands, walks across the room and sits in the window, absorbed in the activities outside. This is usually an indication that he has had enough Reiki, and it is a good time to end the treatment. You may also notice a simultaneous reduction in the flow of energy and may find that you have begun to think about matters unrelated to the treatment.

■ Giving thanks

When finishing a treatment, it is good to remember that you are merely the conduit for this healing energy by putting your hands over your heart and thanking Reiki (we say "Thank you, Reiki" three times). Then, in soft words, internally or out loud, you could thank your animal for opening himself to the process of healing and allowing you to bring Reiki to him. You could stroke your animal briefly before saying goodbye, but often it is better to let your animal be the one to initiate physical contact if he wants it before you leave.

■ After the treatment

Ideally, your animal should be able to rest, if he wants to, after receiving a Reiki treatment. There should be plenty of fresh water available, since the treatment may make him thirsty. If you are treating an animal that is not your own and received any intuitive information during the treatment which you feel would be helpful to share with the animal's person, you may want to convey some or all of it at this time. As we will discuss in Chapter 17, it is not always helpful to share intuitive information received during a treatment. Conveying this information

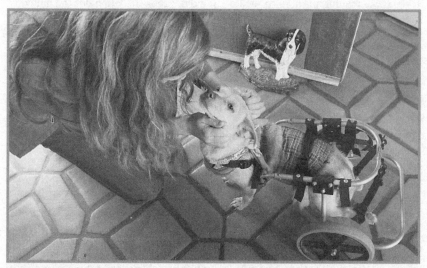

Kathleen thanks Joey for choosing to participate in his own healing process.

A BROKEN HEART IS MENDED

A distinctive thing about Franny, whose story was begun in A Storm of Emotions (page 56), is that she spent all her time at the shelter huddled in her cat bed. She ate and used her litter box only after the shelter closed for the day, when no people were around. When

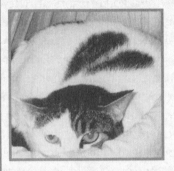

she was lying in her bed, the dark markings on her coat formed a perfect image of a broken heart, the two halves separated by an even white space between them. Many people remarked on how appropriate this marking seemed after she lost her kittens.

After her weekly Reiki treatments and the emotional release accompanying them, Franny would be more open to interactions with people for a few days, but inevitably she would retreat back into her shell. One day I began to wonder if caring for a litter of motherless kittens would be healing for Franny. As fate would have it, the next time I stopped by a litter of very young, orphaned feral kittens had arrived. They were terrified, overwhelmed and not eating.

I asked the staff if I could introduce the kittens to Franny and see if she would care for them. The conventional wisdom is that an adult cat will not care for another's kittens, but I had a strong feeling that this would be an exception. The shelter was willing to give it a try as long as I monitored the situation.

We started with one kitten to see how she did. I took the kitten out to Franny and sat in front of her cage, holding the kitten on my lap with one hand while the other sent Reiki to the situation. Franny seemed to ignore the kitten, but each time it cried, her attention sharpened. Eventually, when I felt she would not harm it, I put the kitten in her cage. The kitten stumbled around, and Franny continued to ignore it. Finally, as closing time approached, I told Franny that this might be her one chance to be a mother and that I would give her five more minutes to make up her mind but then I would have to take the kitten back. Then I held my breath and sent Reiki. About four minutes later the kitten began to cry and, as I reached for it, Franny leaned over and began to lick it. The kitten quieted immediately and snuggled next to Franny.

requires discretion and compassion and is a skill that grows with experience. Always do so carefully, in a way that does not cause distress and that facilitates healing for all concerned.

Often, the healing results of a treatment are apparent immediately, within a few hours or a few days of treatment. Sometimes the healing that has taken place may take some time to be understood.

She tucked the kitten under her chin and rested her head on it. The look on her face was a mixture of stunned incredulousness and utter joy.

The staff joined me, and we stayed with Franny until we felt it was safe to leave the kitten with her overnight. The next morning Franny and the kitten were snuggled together in a picture of complete contentment. We brought the other kittens to Franny; she looked a bit stunned but accepted them all immediately. The staff felt it was important for the kittens to be raised to be comfortable with people so they would not remain feral and could eventually find good homes. So Franny's ability to keep the kittens now hinged on finding a suitable foster home. I went home and once again sent Reiki to the situation.

The next day a kind and generous volunteer, Henry, offered to take Franny home to raise her kittens. A few days later he reported that, incredibly, she was producing milk and was able to nurse all the kittens, even though it had been six weeks or more since her pregnancy had been aborted.

Franny was an excellent mother. Henry interacted with the kittens frequently, and they grew up to be affectionate with people. I continued to visit Franny and offer her Reiki weekly. She was immersed in her role as a mother but never warmed to Henry or to people in general. She let me stroke her and let Henry brush her and take her to the vet, but she declined other interactions, remaining essentially feral in nature. Even at Henry's Franny remained huddled in her bed, coming out only at night after Henry was asleep.

After several months all of the kittens found good homes. I sent Reiki to Franny to help her with the separation from her beloved babies, and she coped well with the loss. However, Franny was still largely feral and uninterested in living as a companion to a human being.

When the kittens went to their new homes, Franny returned to the shelter because Henry was moving away. She had a close call with euthanasia when the shelter was once more overfull, but a volunteer, Mary, stepped in and took her home to live as an outdoor cat. When Mary took Franny outdoors and told her she was free to go, Franny's eyes lit up. She sat beside Mary for a few minutes, looking gratefully up at her, and then disappeared into the foliage. Franny now returns daily to be fed by Mary, sometimes rubbing against her legs and allowing her to stroke her. Since she walked out of her carrier, Franny's broken heart marking has never been seen again, and I believe on an emotional level her heart has healed as well. —*Elizabeth*

■ Frequency and duration of subsequent treatments

As you gain experience, we encourage you to use your intuition and experiment with the duration and frequency of treatments. In the meantime, we have some suggestions to use as a starting point when you begin to treat animals with Reiki. If these ideal guidelines are not possible, in the beginning you should just follow them as closely as the situation permits.

- The healing effects of Reiki treatments build upon one another when they are given close together in time, so, with any condition, it is best to begin with a series of four treatments on consecutive days, if possible.

- For minor health problems, a series of four treatments is optimal, but if it is not possible, once-a-week treatments may be adequate until the problem resolves.

- Serious or chronic problems benefit from a series of four treatments on consecutive days, if possible, followed by at least once- or twice-a-week treatments until the problem resolves.

- For very seriously ill animals or animals with deep spiritual or emotional damage, the optimal approach is to give as much Reiki as possible, particularly at the beginning of a course of treatment. Sometimes daily treatments are necessary to

SUNSHINE MAKES HER PREFERENCE CLEAR

Early in my experience with Reiki, one of the first animals who clearly indicated that she was finished with a treatment was a lovely half-Clydesdale horse

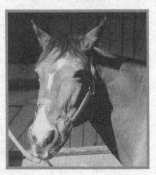

named Sunshine. She was quite smart and accomplished at making human friends at the stable where I had my horse at the time. The first time I gave her a Reiki treatment, she took charge of the treatment, sniffing my hands carefully at the beginning of the treatment and allowing me to place them on her as though doing me a great favor. She dozed and seemed to enjoy the treatment for about 30 minutes. Then she suddenly quivered all over once, looked at me intently and, when I did not move my hands, swatted me soundly with her tail and moved away. It was one of the most unmistakable signals I have received to this day. —*Elizabeth*

reach as deeply into a being as is needed to return him to health. On other occasions, one or two treatments will work apparent miracles, but sometimes it takes a very concerted effort and great dedication to bring about a shift toward health.

- For general energetic balance and health maintenance, every animal will benefit from regular weekly or bi-weekly treatments. Of course, regular daily treatments (of even five or ten minutes) will benefit animals as much as daily self-treatment will benefit you.

■ Accepting the results of a treatment

As Reiki practitioners, we always remember that Reiki does the healing and we are only the conduits for this remarkable healing energy. Of course, the fact that we are present and have the intention of bringing healing is an important part of the process, but it is not our own power that does the healing. And although we may have the best intentions for dramatic cures for every problem, healing does not always mean cure. In retrospect, we can usually see how Reiki brought the healing that was needed most to the situation.

Reiki for Specific Animals

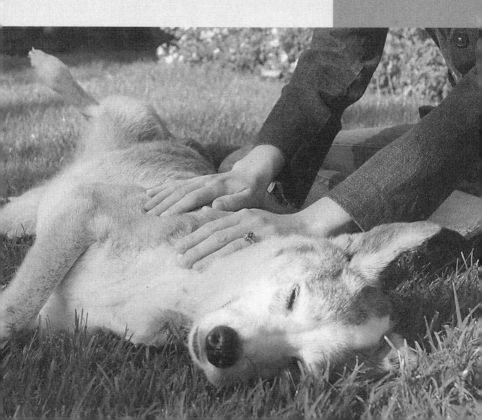

chapter 8
Reiki for Dogs

DOGS, SOCIAL ANIMALS THAT THEY ARE, often take the initiative in any meeting—they'll make that physical connection with you by walking right up to say hi. The best place to give a treatment to your dog may depend upon his size and demeanor. For instance, you can choose a place in the center of a room and sit directly on the floor or, if your dog is large and active, you might want to sit on a chair; this way you won't be knocked over by his exuberance!

Once you are positioned comfortably, you can ask the dog's permission to give him a treatment and let him know that he need only take the Reiki he is comfortable taking. If you let him know this treatment will be at his discretion and under his control, he'll be much more likely to be curious and interested in Reiki.

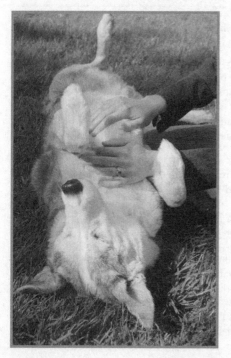

Once you have let your dog know that it's up to him to decide how much Reiki he wants to receive, you can let the energy flow from your hands and allow your dog to approach you in his own way and time. Watch your dog's body language: some dogs quiet down immediately for the entire treatment, right under your hands. Other dogs may pace or circle around you, sitting or lying down periodically until they're able to relax.

Another way to tell whether your dog is accepting the energy is to pay attention to the flow of energy in your hands. If there's a steady flow of energy, your dog is drawing Reiki to himself and beginning to acquaint himself with its benefits. You can continue offering the energy rather than sending it in a coercive way. This is the key to your dog's continued participation and appreciation of his Reiki treatment.

If your dog is feeling playful when you offer him Reiki, try not to encourage him; just remain still and quiet and allow him to sniff you and investigate your hands, which he'll usually do once he senses the energy. Most of the time, when he observes your relaxed behavior and feels the calming sensation of the energy, he'll settle down to rest or sleep. Some dogs may experience a "healing reaction" in the beginning. For example, if your dog has an uncomfortable skin condition, the healing energy may initially cause him to feel itchy and to scratch himself. Just continue sending Reiki and this will pass, and he'll eventually relax, actually feeling relief from his symptoms. (See page 16 for further information about healing reactions.)

How a dog "accepts" a Reiki treatment is unique for each dog,

DAKOTA: "REIKI TEACHER EXTRAORDINAIRE"

Dakota has been my dog companion for the last 13 years, and has been asking for and receiving Reiki on a daily basis since I first learned Level 1 Reiki back in 1998. In fact, he's really my inspiration for pursuing my career as an animal Reiki teacher and practitioner. When I first learned Reiki, my teachers emphasized self-treatment and human treatment. I was so excited with the results I'd seen in my own health issues that I began doing self-treatment every night once I learned Level 1.

Dakota has always liked to be in the room wherever I am, but I noticed a change in his behavior once I learned Reiki. Every time I'd begin doing a self-treatment (I'd usually sit on the couch in the living room), he'd come over to me and lie down right across my feet in a most awkward position. It was as if he were trying to absorb the "run-off" energy from my treatment on myself!

After a few nights of this behavior, a light bulb went on in my head: I realized that he might be asking me for some Reiki! So the next time he came over to lay across my feet, I got off the couch, sat down on the floor and just put my hands on him. My hands really heated up and he immediately stretched out flat and relaxed, took a deep sigh and closed his eyes. I realized that he was taking as much Reiki as I and the other humans whom I had worked on did.

and even for the same dog in different treatments. Some dogs will come directly to you, climb onto your lap and fall into a "Reiki sleep" almost immediately. Some dogs may lie down behind you to rest, feeling more comfortable if they're facing in the other direction. Other dogs prefer to settle down 10 to 15 feet away, looking at you, or positioning the areas of their bodies that need healing closest to you.

Many dogs will come to you, resting directly under your hands for a treatment. Sometimes they're more comfortable if you gently stroke them with one hand while your other hand is resting quietly on them, sending Reiki. Other dogs prefer to be lightly scratched with the fingers of your hand while you keep your palms resting quietly on them, sending Reiki. Just experiment until you find the position(s) that your dog likes best and where he's able to relax fully into his treatment.

▬ Overview of the treatment

The approach Always begin by asking your dog to take only the amount of energy he finds comfortable and continue this respect-

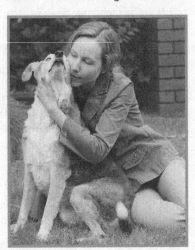

And even more extraordinary, it appeared that he not only understood what Reiki was but also sought it out on his own for healing.

This realization was life changing for me. I had always had a deep empathetic connection with animals, and suddenly I realized I could give them the gift of Reiki. What followed was several years of trial and error with many species of animals in many places . . . many lessons learned from these animal teachers and, eventually, the motivation to write this book.

I have the deepest gratitude to my dearest dog friend and teacher Dakota for his patience in my learning process and his willingness to show me the way. These days, he often serves as a teacher for my Level 1 students, and he also served as the model for most of the photos illustrating this chapter, a job he took on with great gusto. Thank you, my wonderful boy! —*Kathleen*

GAINING YOUR DOG'S
COOPERATION AND ACCEPTANCE

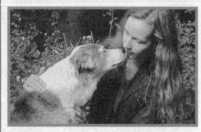

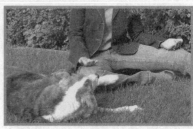

Before starting a treatment, ask your dog, "Would you like a Reiki treatment?" Then ask him to take only the amount of Reiki he finds comfortable. This is an important step. If you forget and just begin the treatment, your dog may not want to participate.

If your dog wants a treatment, he'll let you know through his body language and the flow of energy in your hands. As soon as Kathleen asks Dakota for permission, he immediately lies down and looks at her with interest: a definite "Yes, please!"

ful attitude throughout the treatment. Use your intuition and observations of your dog's body language to determine whether to give hands-on or distant Reiki and to tell when he has had enough Reiki. Just "offer" Reiki and let the dog take as much as he finds comfortable.

Treating from a distance If your dog is more comfortable taking Reiki from a distance, allow him this space. The most important thing is to let him move around and determine the conditions of treatment. Your intention, your dog's acceptance, and the energetic essence of Reiki—not the proximity and placement of your hands—create an effective healing treatment.

Basic body positions Begin on the shoulders and move down the body. If your dog is relaxed and dozing, you may not want to disturb him by moving your hands or trying to do both sides of his body: just use the positions that work best for your dog. Reiki can be done from only one position if that's what is most comfortable for him.

Extra positions For mental/emotional healing, try placing one hand on his chest and the other hand on the head, or on his back between his shoulders, to give him a mental healing. Many animals prefer not to have your hands on their heads so use your intuition to see what your dog's preference is.

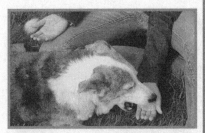

Here you can see Dakota yawning. This "Reiki yawn" is a common way animals show acceptance of the energy as they relax and enjoy the treatment. Deep sighs are another common sign that Reiki is doing its work.

Finishing the treatment Thank Reiki for the healing and your dog for his participation. You may want to spend some time petting or massaging him if he's open to it. This is a wonderful time to bond!

(see Chapters 4 and 5 for further information)

▬ Treating from a distance

Many dogs like to receive the entire treatment from a few feet away (see picture 1 on page 82). Sometimes, they move around, coming to your hands and moving away and perhaps resting. They may do this several times. You can trust that Reiki is effec-tive even when your hands aren't directly on your dog's body.

Experiment with the way your dog likes to receive his Reiki treatment. In picture 2 on page 82, you can see another alternative: one hand on, one off. Sometimes your dog will position himself so that you can't reach him with both hands. In this case, you don't need to move him or move closer to him; just place the hand closest to him lightly on him and rest your other hand in your lap.

You can treat your dog from across the room or yard—and even greater distances—when you learn Level 2 Reiki. Notice the relaxation Dakota shows in picture 3 on page 82; you can see that even without direct hand contact, he's very relaxed and accepting of the Reiki treatment.

To finish the treatment, thank your dog for his acceptance and participation. In picture 4 on page 82, Kathleen spends a few moments saying, "Thank you, Dakota! Good boy!"

▬ Hands-on treatment

Let your dog decide how and where to receive Reiki. If your

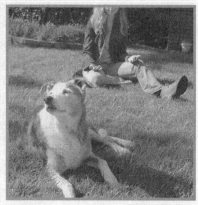

1. Many dogs prefer treatment from a few feet away.

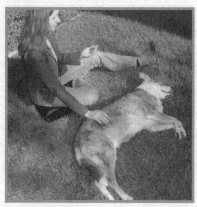

2. Some like one hand on and one hand off.

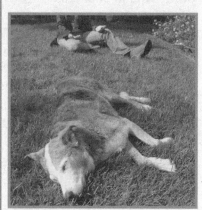

3. With Level 2 Reiki, you can treat your dog from greater distances.

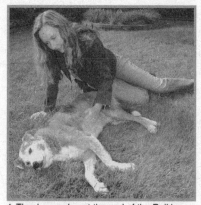

4. Thank your dog at the end of the Reiki treatment.

dog starts a treatment in a standing position, he'll probably soon relax and lie down.

Sometimes when small dogs want Reiki, they climb onto your lap, where you can do the entire treatment from one or two positions. They'll often lie down once they relax into the treatment.

WHEN YOUR DOG IS LYING DOWN

If your dog chooses hands-on Reiki, the shoulders are a great place to let him first feel the sensation of the energy (picture 1 below). Rest your hands lightly, without pressure, on your dog's body. If your dog looks uncertain or uncomfortable at any time when you place your hands on him or move them, you can do the entire treatment from one position or from a distance. Similarly, if you sense that moving your hands will disturb your dog's relaxation or cause him to become restless, you can stay in one position for the whole treatment.

As you continue, move your hands down his body toward his hind end. Always rest your hands lightly without pressure. If you

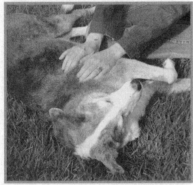

1. If your dog chooses hands-on Reiki, the shoulders are a great place to start.

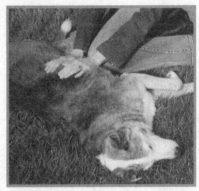

2. Continue treatment by gently moving your hands down his body toward his hind end.

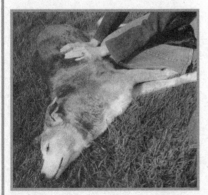

3. Be flexible with your hand positions if he moves around.

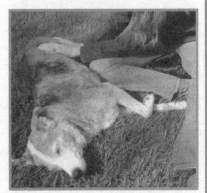

4. Treating the hind end near the tail is one good way to finish a treatment.

sense it's more comfortable for your dog, you can hold your hands a few inches from his body. If your dog is comfortable with hands-on Reiki, you can place your hands on or near his side (see picture 2 on page 83), or place your hands closer to the spine as you move your hands down his body—it depends on the position your dog has chosen in relation to you and where it's most comfortable for you to rest your hands.

Continue moving your hands toward his hind end, resting your hands gently on your dog, and being flexible if he moves around

REIKI TREATMENT WHILE YOUR DOG IS SITTING OR STANDING

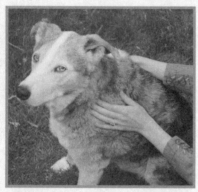

1. Lightly rest your hands on your dog's shoulders to start.

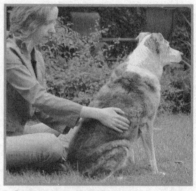

2. Continue down the back, on either side of the spine, to your dog's hind end.

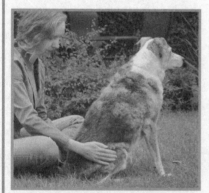

3. Finish the treatment on the hind end, if your dog is comfortable with your hands there.

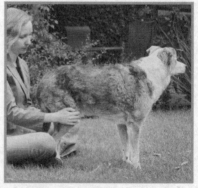

4. Your dog may stand and put a part of his body in your hands when he wants Reiki there.

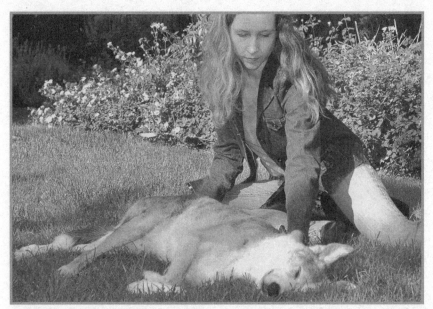
This is an optional final position for giving a Reiki treatment while your dog is lying down.

(see picture 3 on page 83). Your dog's comfort is more important than retaining the exact hand position.

You may end the session by treating your dog's hind end near the tail. This is one good way to finish a treatment (see picture 4 on page 83). As you can see from this series, you needn't be concerned about treating both sides of your dog, who may roll over to receive Reiki on a particular spot. It's possible to give a complete treatment on just one side, moving from shoulder to hind end, or even from one position. Reiki will go where it's needed.

After moving down your dog's sides from shoulder to hind end, this is another great way to finish a treatment: with one hand at his head, the other at the base of his tail (see above). Offering Reiki simultaneously from both ends of the spine will give your dog a feeling of energetic balance.

WHEN YOUR DOG IS SITTING OR STANDING

The shoulders are also a good place to start when your dog is sitting or standing (see picture 1 on page 84). It's a comfortable place for most dogs to feel the energy and your hands as you begin the treatment. Lightly rest

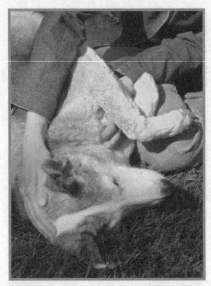

Placing one hand on your dog's chest and the other hand on the head is a good way to focus on emotional healing.

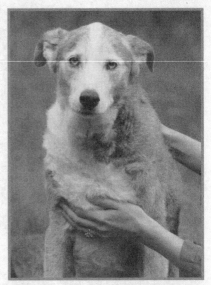

Another way to focus on emotional healing is to place one hand on your dog's chest and the other on the back between the shoulders.

your hands on your dog. Soon he'll begin to relax.

If your dog is comfortable with the movement of your hands, you can continue to move down his back to his hind end, on either side of his spine (see picture 2 on page 84).

Finish the treatment on his hind end, if your dog is comfortable with your hands there (see picture 3 on page 84). Some dogs with arthritis or hip dysplasia may find the energy too intense so close to the joint. In this case, you could try the entire treatment from the shoulder position, from a few inches away or from a

short distance. You may need to experiment to see what is best for your dog. Reiki will flow like a magnet where it's needed, even if your hands aren't directly over the areas in need.

He may stand up and put a part of his body in your hands when he particularly wants Reiki there (see picture 4 on page 84).

MENTAL AND EMOTIONAL HEALING

Sometimes as you treat your dog, you may get the sense that he needs healing for an emotional problem. Let your intuition and your dog's preference guide you. The two positions pictured above are good ways to focus on emotional healing. One approach is to place one hand on his chest and the other hand on his head, if he's comfortable with it, or, alternatively, one hand on his chest and the other on his back between his shoulders.

Sometimes your dog will offer you his belly, and some dogs love this position. Don't worry about the exact position your hands are in; just find a place to put your hands that's comfortable for him.

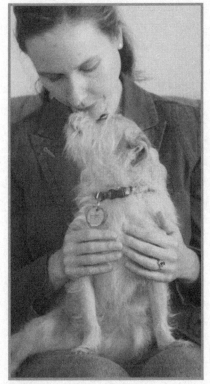
Colby accepts hands-on Reiki.

Smaller dogs with emotional issues may even take Reiki on your lap, just like Colby, a terrier mix. Colby was surrendered by her first owners and was adopted by Emily and her family. At first, she was a bundle of nerves. She shook constantly and howled and cried if left alone. Over time, with the love and support of her new family, she became less fearful, but she still hated being left by her people. Colby's increasing confidence, however, was demonstrated in her choice of how to receive a Reiki treatment. She actually chose to be in Kathleen's lap for hands-on Reiki, rather than receiving it from a distance, as many fearful dogs prefer. She soaked up the energy like a true Reiki sponge.

TREATING YOUR DOG'S LEGS

The positions below are useful for injuries or conditions that affect the legs and feet. However, only use these positions if your dog is comfortable with them and has consented to hands-on Reiki. First, make sure your dog is in a comfortable position, such as lying down. Gently try the following hand positions:

The front leg: Gently place one hand on the elbow and rest the leg in your other hand.

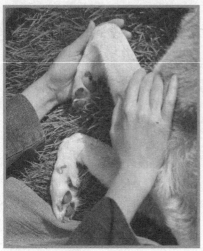
Reiki on the front leg

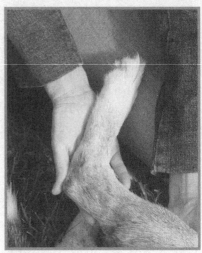
Reiki on the hind leg

For the hind leg: Start with both hands at the hip. You can then move your hands toward the hind paw, resting one hand on the upper leg and placing the lower leg in your other hand.

chapter 9

Reiki for Cats

■ Cats crave Reiki

KNOWN FOR THEIR INDEPENDENT NATURE, cats prefer Reiki on their own terms. Like many animals, if they sense that you're trying to coerce their participation in the treatment, they'll have no part in it. If you begin a treatment with a cat by offering him the healing energy of Reiki and asking him to take only as much as he wants, he'll generally be very open to receiving it. Before you start, it can be helpful to detach yourself from any expectations you may have about the treatment and to center yourself emotionally. The best way to gain your

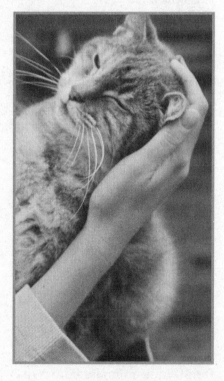

cat's trust and acceptance of Reiki is to find a comfortable place in the room at a bit of a distance from him, and just sit quietly, letting him know that you'll be offering him only as much Reiki as he feels comfortable receiving.

By offering Reiki to your cat from a short distance, you can give him a chance to evaluate it in his own way and in as much time as he needs to become comfortable with it. When he doesn't feel pressured or coerced, you'll usually find that your cat quickly learns to enjoy and seek out Reiki healing and to appreciate the treatments as a special time between the two of you.

A Reiki treatment will start as soon as you allow the Reiki energy to begin flowing from your hands. Your cat will sense the presence of the

DR. MU SHU

My lovely black-and-white cat, Mu Shu, arrived home one day with blood caked on her ear from an encounter with the local feline bully. The next day her ear was swollen and she clearly wasn't feeling well, so I took her in to our veterinarian to have him take a look at her ear. He shaved it and found that the bully had bitten all the way through her ear and had torn almost a half-inch slit in it. Since there is relatively little blood flow to a cat's ear, he was concerned that it wouldn't heal well and she'd have a permanently collapsed ear. He gave her a shot of antibiotics and sent us home.

Over the next few days Mu Shu shadowed me everywhere, and each time I sat down she'd jump up on my lap for Reiki. I was exceptionally busy and engrossed in my work and responded largely on automatic pilot to Mu Shu's requests for Reiki, complying with her wish but with my mind mostly still on other matters at hand. For several days I did everything one-handed, working at the computer, reading, talking on the phone, and sometimes even eating, while the other hand, at her insistence, was glued to Mu Shu with the Reiki "tap" turned full on.

On the fifth day, while Mu Shu was happily ensconced on my lap and hooked up to Reiki, I looked down at her ear and noticed that there was only a tiny pinhead-size scab left to show where the injury had been, with no scar or other sign of her recent, very nasty injury. Mu Shu, veteran of Reiki healing that she is, knew exactly how to get the healing she felt she needed and took charge of obtaining it without a lot of conscious involvement on my part—I just followed Dr. Mu Shu's excellent treatment plan. —*Elizabeth*

energy immediately and will often come to investigate. For instance, he may come directly over to your hands and sniff them, or he may approach you and look at you very intently or curiously. You'll be able to tell whether he's open to the treatment by his body language and by the energy flow through your hands. (See Chapter 4 for more information about how to understand your animal's body language and the flow of energy in your hands.)

The way a cat receives a treatment is different for each cat and for each treatment. Some cats will curl up in their beds or head for their favorite nap places and fall into a deep sleep, even twitching and running in kitty dreams. Other cats will crawl up onto your lap or even onto your chest and begin purring loudly. At this point the cat may want you to give him a hands-on treatment and if you feel this is the case, you could try placing one hand on your cat and see what his response to this is. If he accepts this, you could add your other hand and see how he responds again. Some cats prefer to move around during the treatment, perhaps first settling down to sleep, then coming over to sniff your hands, then lying in front of you for a few minutes, then rubbing against your back, then sleeping across from you, or finally crawling into your lap for hands-on Reiki during the last few minutes of the treatment.

Your cat may do any of these things alone or in combinations, or he may do something else altogether that seems appropriate to him. There's no need to worry about how your cat accepts Reiki. If he moves around during the treatment, he'll be receiving Reiki very effectively regardless, so there's no reason to feel he's "missing" something. Keep in mind that your cat's preferences can change even from one treatment to the next.

When there's more than one cat in a household, Reiki can be offered to all the cats together as a group. Group treatment is very effective and can be convenient for people with more than one cat who don't have time to offer separate treatments. Sometimes the cats will decide who goes first and take turns receiving their treatments. On other occasions they'll crowd around you as you give the treatment, and you may end up with each hand on a different cat, or a cat under one hand and the others clustered nearby, all absorbing the energy.

When cats have had enough Reiki, they'll let you know. For

TREATING MULTIPLE CATS

It's possible to do hands-on Reiki with multiple cats at once, and it's best to open up treatment to all your animals so that no one feels left out or gets jealous. In the photo to the right, Bobby receives a hands-on treatment and Sammi joins in. Kathleen doesn't have to place her hands directly on Sammi—she's absorbing the energy just by being nearby. Remember: The energy will go where it needs to go. Your cats will let you know how they want the treatment by where they position themselves as you offer Reiki. You will be able to tell they are receiving Reiki by their relaxation.

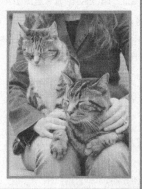

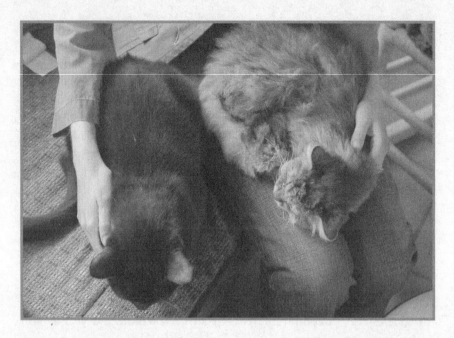

instance, they may wake up, yawn, stretch, get a drink of water, become absorbed in another activity, leave the room or go outside. The flow of Reiki through your hands may also taper off at about the same time. You may even feel the flow of energy taper off in your hands while the cat's still sleeping, in which case you can quietly leave the room, allowing your cat to enjoy the deep sleep that can accompany a Reiki treatment.

▬ Overview of the treatment

The approach Always begin by asking permission, letting your cat know that he need only take the energy he wants. Watch your cat's body language to discover how he prefers a treatment. Remember to not push Reiki on your feline friend: just offer it and see what he chooses.

Treating from a distance Most cats prefer Reiki from a distance. Your cat will probably settle nearby (perhaps even resting against you) or several feet away during the treatment. There's often movement during the treatment as well: your cat may come to you and smell your hands, and then go across the room and settle peacefully in his bed for the duration of the treatment. Let your cat decide how close he wants to be for his treatment.

SIMON: BREATHING A BIT EASIER

The first time I met Simon, he was having a tough day. Simon suffers from chronic asthma, and some days it's very hard for him to breathe. I had come to visit BrightHaven animal sanctuary that day to offer Reiki to one of my favorite cats there, Crystal. She was approaching the end of her life, and has since experienced a peaceful passing with lots of Reiki support. As I finished my treatment with Crystal, a shiny, beautiful black cat ran into the room and literally threw himself on me, rubbing his head all over my arms, legs and sides. He meowed impatiently, as if he wanted me to begin his treatment immediately!

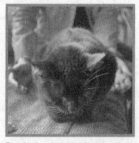

By placing her hands near, but not *on*, Simon, Kathleen can offer him Reiki without disturbing his relaxation.

I sat on the floor and he settled his body into my lap so that my hands were over his lung area. My hands heated up immediately, and he took a deep and rumbling sigh, settling in for the treatment. About halfway through the treatment, he had a terrible coughing episode: his nose sounded terribly stuffy and began to run, and it sounded as if he couldn't catch his breath. After a moment, it was as if the coughing episode had cleared his lungs: he took a deep breath and fell asleep. I continued the treatment for nearly an hour, eventually having to end it because of an appointment I had elsewhere. It was difficult to get him to leave my lap: he clung to me with his paws and meowed plaintively. I dearly wished I could have stayed longer! When I got home, I put him on my distant client list for the animals who receive regular group distant treatments.

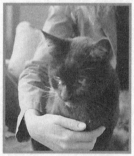

Simon backs into Kathleen's hands so that she can place her hand on his chest.

From that day on, whenever I visit BrightHaven, I can always count on Simon to find me at some point during the day. He always runs into the room and bounds up into my lap with joy and expectation. He seems to find tremendous comfort from Reiki for his asthma, although he does seem to experience a coughing episode each treatment, a kind of "healing reaction." Although these healing reactions look a bit uncomfortable, he always looks so much better and more comfortable by the end of the treatment. —*Kathleen*

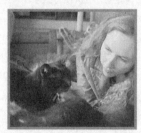

Kathleen thanks Simon for participating in the Reiki treatment.

GRADY: AN AMAZING RECOVERY

When I first met Grady, he had a high fever and was very lethargic. He was on his way to the vet, and I just barely had time for a quick Reiki treatment before his appointment. He was very open to the Reiki, and although he had been unable to relax for some time, fell fast asleep during the treatment.

Once at the vet's, Grady was diagnosed with pyothorax, or infection of the pleural space between the lungs and the chest wall. He was immediately

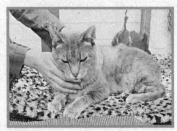

Grady settles in for a "Reiki nap." Rather than disturb his relaxation, Kathleen does the entire treatment from this position.

placed in an oxygen tank and pronounced not strong enough for surgery. His prognosis was not good.

I continued to send daily distant treatments to him, feeling an incredible amount of energy flow each time. Amazingly, he recovered his strength enough to have surgery. I sent him Reiki the day of his surgery as well, and for several consecutive days after. The surgery was a great success, and he has now fully recovered. Today, he's such a big, strong, handsome boy, you'd never know how close he came to death. Although not always open to hands-on attention from people, he happily accepts hands-on Reiki from me whenever I come to visit. —*Kathleen*

Basic body positions Cats are generally smaller than dogs, so usually one or two hand positions during treatment will suffice. Cats often enjoy having your hands on both sides of their body, one hand on the chest and the other on the back, or your hands on their back or hind end. Be sensitive to your cat's preferences.

Extra positions Occasionally, when your cat has a specific health issue, he may place the affected part of his body into your hands, for example, resting his head or a paw in your hands during treatment. Just remain flexible, and allow your cat to show you the areas that need hands-on Reiki.

Finishing the treatment When your cat's finished with his treatment, he may come up and thank you with a nudge or a kiss. Before he leaves to resume his day, thank him for accepting the treatment and perhaps spend a few minutes petting him and letting him know how much you appreciate his participation.

(see Chapters 4 and 5 for further information)

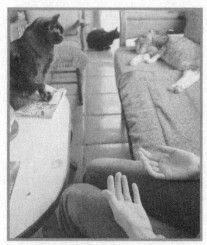
Place yourself in the room and allow the cats who want Reiki to approach.

ther away. They feel the energy and are deciding whether they want a treatment and finding their comfort zone—the distance at which they prefer to receive Reiki. When you're patient and allow the animal to come to you, they'll sometimes choose hands-on Reiki.

Treatment from a distance

To begin the treatment, place yourself in the room and allow the cats who want Reiki to approach. Cats prefer the choice of how to receive Reiki. In the picture above, notice that several cats are relaxed and remain nearby; others have moved far-

Hands-on treatment

Cats often move around at the beginning of a Reiki treatment, finding the position in your hands that is best for them, before settling in for a "Reiki nap." Let the cat move, moving your hands with her. Start with your hands on her shoulders and see where your cat leads you.

Note: Don't try to force your cat to settle. Be patient and let her choose how the treatment will unfold (picture 1 on page 96).

BOBBY AND LINDA

When Bobby arrived at BrightHaven, he was very sick and not eating. Although he has improved tremendously over time, he still suffers from chronic mouth problems. A very sweet and affectionate boy, Bobby loves his Reiki treatments. He's also benefiting from regular acupuncture treatments.

Linda was a feral who one day brought her mate and five kittens into Gail's home to stay. Although very frightened of people at first, she's now extremely loving to people and always ready to sit on a lap. Linda doesn't want to be left out of the group during Reiki treatments at BrightHaven, and always places herself directly on my lap or very close by to be a part of things. Her chronic rhinitis is also helped with homeopathy and acupuncture. —*Kathleen*

If your cat continues to move periodically during the treatment, let yourself use the hand positions that your cat chooses, in the order she wants them used. Don't worry about the number and order of hand positions, just follow your cat's lead. You may end up treating from only one or two positions, or your cat may

SAMMI'S HANDS-ON TREATMENT

Sammi lived as a feral where BrightHaven was formerly located. One day, of her own accord, she decided to move into the house. Very skinny and frightened of humans when she first arrived, her transformation has been amazing! She's now the most loveable, affectionate and easy-going girl, always up for a hands-on Reiki treatment. —*Kathleen*

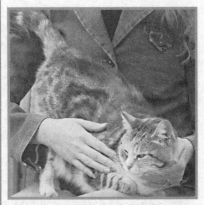

1. Sammi settles in for her Reiki treatment.

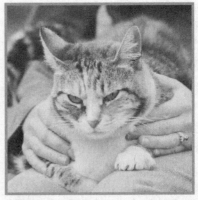

2. Kathleen starts the treatment at Sammi's shoulders.

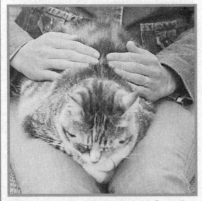

3. Kathleen moves her hands down Sammi's body on either side of her spine.

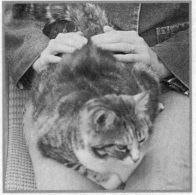

4. The Reiki treatment ends at the base of Sammi's spine.

OLIVER, THE CAT WITH A HEART OF GOLD

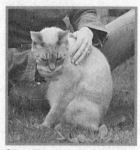

Oliver, like most cats, loves this position: one hand on the chest, the other on the shoulders.

I first met Oliver at BrightHaven through his celebrity status. His story of survival against all odds was featured on an episode of the television series, *Animal Miracles*. Oliver has only three legs due to his brush with death (i.e., predators) several years ago, but the way he gets around you'd never know it! He has the most beautiful blue eyes that seem to look right into your very soul. Oliver's special gift is his compassion and love for others. He adopts the animals at BrightHaven who are most needy, often the ones approaching the end of their lives, and becomes their best companion to the end.

Oliver has accepted Reiki since the very first treatment, as if he and Reiki had been old friends for many years. He's so relaxed and peaceful during treatments; it's as if he understands that Reiki is healing him exactly in the ways he needs it most, and he's grateful to just lay back and soak up the energy. To me, it feels as if my heart gets very big and filled with love when I offer Reiki to Oliver; I feel it must be the energy flowing to Oliver's heart, to his kindness and compassion that know no bounds! It's as if Reiki is supporting Oliver in his mission to be there for the animals who need it most. —*Kathleen*

continually move your hands over her head, body and legs. Reiki will go where it needs to go.

Sometimes cats do settle, falling into a deep sleep for the duration of the treatment. In these cases, there are several body positions you can consider: Start at the shoulders (picture 2, page 96). Move your hands down the body, on either side of the spine (picture 3, page 96). Finish at the base of the spine (picture 4, page 96).

Remember when your cat is settled or sleeping, he is deeply absorbing the Reiki treatment. If moving your hands disturbs his rest or causes him to become concerned or uncomfortable, then it is better to just stay put and do the whole treatment from the position that seems most comfortable for him

chapter 10

Reiki for Horses

HORSES ARE ENERGETICALLY SENSITIVE creatures with a curious nature; they'll immediately sense the energy you offer them, probably coming up to your hands directly to investigate. Try to let go of your expectations for the treatment, and let them determine how things will go; your treatment will be much more successful when you let them approach you, rather than the other way around.

Before you begin the treatment, make sure the horse is in a place where he's comfortable, free to move around, and where you'll not be disturbed. It's possible to treat a horse while he's in a pasture with other horses, but more often than not in this situation, the alpha horse will demand his share of Reiki first, often not allowing other horses to approach. You may end up treating all the horses at once and possibly from a considerable distance. Reiki works from a distance, and you can treat several horses at the same time, but it's better, especially when you're first learning, to treat your horse separately, as he and you will be better able to relax fully and you'll be better able to focus on his

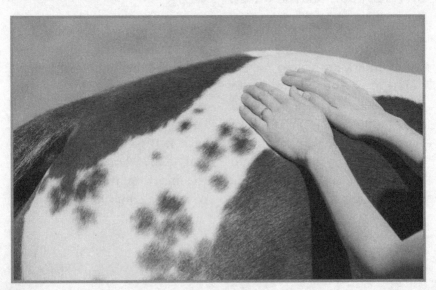

TESS: BLUE RIBBON LADY

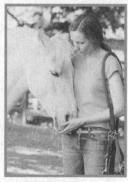

Tess and Kathleen.

One of my Reiki clients is Tess, a dainty and beautiful pony with a kind heart. She teaches little children how to ride. She is patient, kind and gentle with even the youngest riders. It would be impossible to count the dozens of blue ribbons she has won for little kids at their first shows. She has truly touched and enriched many children's lives.

Tess accepts her Reiki treatments as she accepts life—with grace and dignity, and a certain gentleness of spirit that's hard to describe, but anyone who knows her knows what I mean. Tess' chronic health challenge is her digestion. I always know when her stomach is bothering her because during the Reiki treatment, she'll lay down right next to me and roll. Then she'll lift her head from rolling and just lay there, looking at me. By the end of the treatment, she feels much better: she'll get up, take a big sigh and shake herself off. —*Kathleen*

responses and your own intuition about how he's accepting the treatment.

A separate paddock or corral is a perfect place to give a treatment. Here, your horse will be able to relax and accept the Reiki from the distance that makes him most comfortable, without distractions from other horses or people. Reiki will work through stable blankets, fly sheets, bandages and wraps, so whatever covering makes him most comfortable is the best way to start. Enter his paddock, asking his permission and letting him know that he need only take the energy that he wants, and that you won't be coercing his participation. Stand 10 to 15 feet away from your horse at first, with your hands lowered at your sides, and just ask Reiki to begin flowing. Watch for signs of acceptance such as your horse approaching you to lick your hands, lowering his head, cocking a back leg, licking and chewing, or settling in for a nap.

Every horse is different, as are subsequent treatments of the same horse, so it's important always to begin each treatment this way from a distance, even if you know your horse very well and treat him regularly. It's very common for horses to come and go from your hands, and you should allow them to do so, not following them when they walk away. Just as you may feel the ebb and flow of the energy in your hands, there's an "ebb and flow" in the way they may take the treatment. They may move close to you or away from you, settling against your hands and then moving away, then coming back and so on, and this pattern may be repeated several times during the treatment.

This being said, horses often enjoy hands-on treatments. In this case, they'll come to you, settle quietly and nap for the entire session. If the horse is open to hands-on treatment, a series of hand positions (demonstrated in the pictures that follow) will work very well in healing and balancing his energy, as well as giving you feedback about issues your horse may be facing. Follow your intuition as well as the horse's behavior to determine areas that may need healing. Your horse may turn his body or actually back or sidestep certain parts of his body directly into

SHAWNEE

I have always loved horses and ridden many throughout my life, but Shawnee is my most special horse companion—he's the first horse I can call my very own. I found him about four years ago. The horse I had been riding and sponsoring was being retired by his person and sent to a retirement farm several hours away. It was heartbreaking for me to say goodbye, but I realized it was time for a new chapter in my "horsey life"; I was ready to have a horse of my own. I began giving distant Reiki treatments to this situation, trusting that the right horse would find me, and that I would know him when I saw him.

A few months later, unexpectedly, I was introduced to Shawnee when visiting a new barn where Elizabeth had recently moved her horse. His person had become ill, was unable to care for him, and was anxious to sell him. In the first day I spent with him, just grooming him (his feet were overgrown, he had rain rot and his mane and tail were matted) and spending time with him as he grazed, I was very impressed with his gentle nature and the serene energy he had. A few days later, I returned again but he had been moved (without my knowledge) to a different place at the ranch. As I searched the pasture for him, I suddenly heard a loud whinny behind me. I turned to look and there he was, across the ranch, staring intently at me, both ears pricked forward with anticipation. I couldn't believe it—after only a few hours together, he recognized me; it was as if he had already chosen me!

your hands for Reiki healing. He may stomp a foot that is uncomfortable, shift his weight away from a sore leg, or even lift and dramatically stretch his leg or even his entire spine, depending on where he needs healing. He may offer you his head or chest, standing very still and quiet, for emotional healing. And when he's finished with the treatment, he'll probably thank you with a kiss, a push of his nose, or a loud snort before moving away from you to return to more everyday equine behaviors.

■ Overview of the treatment

The approach   Always ask permission first, letting your horse know that he need only take the energy he wants. Most horses appreciate a verbal greeting and a pat before beginning.

Treating from a distance   Begin your treatment at a distance and let your horse determine how far away you should be when giving a treatment. Don't follow him if he moves away, just continue allowing the energy to flow.

We spent several more days together; I even rode him in the arena and on nearby trails. He was so willing and sweet, I realized that this was the horse for me. Unfortunately, the vet check showed that he had advanced arthritis in three legs. He had been used as a cow horse and reiner since a very young age and had the arthritis to prove it. In spite of this news, I bought him and began giving him Reiki treatments three to five times a week.

With regular Reiki treatments after each ride, I brought him slowly back into a training program. A Western horse his whole life, he now switched to dressage training and took to it easily. Within several months, he was completely sound and in terrific shape, his coat shining like a brand-new penny. I was careful to not overdo it, and people who watched us together couldn't believe that he had any arthritis at all. He loved his Reiki treatments and came to expect them each time he was ridden. As my Reiki business expanded at the barn, he watched me patiently as I gave Reiki treatments to the other horses, waiting for his turn. In time, I began to bring students to the barn to practice Reiki with Shawnee. Occasionally, this would be the first time the person had been around a horse, and Shawnee was gentle, patient and, as always, a wonderful Reiki teacher.

Recently, I've decided to retire Shawnee from riding. I think he's earned a life of leisure in the pasture, with lots of love, grooming, walks and grazing. But I know he won't mind teaching a few Reiki students now and again. —*Kathleen*

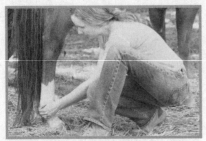

When treating a horse's leg, squat nearby and to the side.

Basic body positions Begin on one shoulder, alternate sides, and move down the back on either side of the spine. Finish on the hind end.

Extra positions You may add the legs, focusing on the joints, and, if your horse asks for it, hand positions on the head.

Finishing the treatment Thank your horse for his participation in the treatment and, if he likes, spend a few moments with him for pats or a little massage.

(see Chapters 4 and 5 for further information)

▬ Treating from a distance

Many horses prefer receiving Reiki from a distance; Reiki is just as effective when given at a distance as it is when given hands-on. Because Reiki is energy, it can easily travel across this distance, provided you have the intention

to offer it and your horse is willing to accept the treatment. Because horses are in general very sensitive to energy and intelligent, you will usually find that your horse shows you very clearly that he's feeling and enjoying the energy.

As with any treatment, it's important to begin by asking permission. As you can see in picture 1 on page 103, Kodiak is very interested in grazing and has thus ignored Kathleen's presence in the pasture up to this point.

Once she begins offering Reiki to him, Kodiak feels the energy immediately. In this case, he stops his grazing (the energy is even more interesting to him than eating) and walks directly

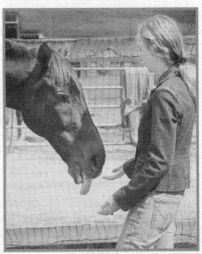

Swenson deeply relaxes into a Reiki treatment.

TREATING FROM A DISTANCE

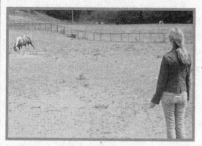

1. Kathleen asks Kodiak for permission to give him a Reiki treatment.

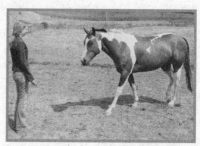

2. Kodiak senses the Reiki and approaches Kathleen's hands.

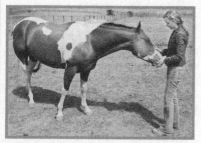

3. During treatment, Kodiak nuzzles her hands, perhaps enjoying the energy.

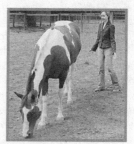

4. Kodiak allows Kathleen to focus Reiki on his hind end.

up to Kathleen's hands (picture 2 above).

Kodiak is just a baby and very sensitive. He continues to mouth Kathleen's hands for a few minutes (picture 3 above). Perhaps the energy tickles his mouth because he often shows this behavior at the beginning of Reiki treatments.

After several moments, he relaxes and grazes again, but this time he stays closer to Kathleen, still aware of the treatment and engaged with the energy. He eventually turns his body around so that the energy is focused on his hind end (picture 4 above).

Sometimes you may find yourself in a time and place where Reiki is greatly needed. One such example happened on a fall day when Elizabeth was at the stable with her horses. She observed a difficult situation unfolding: A couple who had

KODIAK: BABY BLUE EYES

Kodiak and I found each other in February 2005. Recently turned four, he's truly a "1,000-pound toddler." His attention span is really short, everything goes in his mouth, and he loves to say "No!" and see what happens. It's a new and exciting experience for me to be a part of his growing up. I've been able

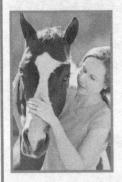

to watch his baby teeth fall out and to be there to watch him learn new things every day; he's so smart and curious, he absorbs every new experience with passion. The sparkling and vibrant energy he gives off is infectious to everyone around him.

Kodiak takes Reiki the way he lives life—he absorbs it with 110 percent enthusiasm, and then after a few minutes, he's ready for the next adventure. A few days after I brought him home, Kodiak stumbled into a fence and cut his nose. After the veterinarian stitched it up, I offered him Reiki to help him heal. As the Reiki began flowing, he yawned repeatedly, closed his eyes and lowered his head to sleep. After about 15 minutes, he woke up and looked at me as if to say, "OK, I'm done. What's next?" Subsequent Reiki treatments are the same: short but powerful. As long as I continue to ask permission and allow him to determine the duration of the treatment, Kodiak is a very willing "Reiki sponge." —*Kathleen*

been boarding a mare and her foal there were trying to move them to another facility. The foal hadn't been handled much since birth and was very wary of humans.

The husband caught the mother and loaded her in the trailer, and the wife was trying to catch the foal. The foal was calling to his mother and becoming increasingly panicky by the minute. He slipped past the wife and got out into a big open area of an acre or so and ran around wildly in a full-blown panic. The mother was screaming for her foal and rearing up in the trailer, trying to get out and go to her foal. The couple began to chase the foal around, increasing his panic. After several minutes, everyone involved—the horse, her foal and the people—were extremely upset, and it looked as if there could be no peaceful resolution to the situation. Elizabeth mentally drew the Level 2 Reiki symbols and let energy flow to the situation.

Within minutes the situation began to de-escalate. The couple stopped chasing the foal, the mother stopped screaming and rearing, and the foal calmed enough so that the husband was able to get a lead line then a halter on him, and lead him into the trailer with his mother. As they drove away safely, Elizabeth was grateful once again for Reiki's gentle but powerful action.

■ Hands-on treatment

Sixty minutes is a good average duration for a hands-on full-body treatment. Some suggested hand positions are detailed here, but these are only recommended; remember, your horse's preference is the most important consideration when you do hands-on treatment. If a position is uncomfortable for him, your horse will show you this by moving away from you if you touch a sensitive area; allow your horse to determine the duration and course of the treatment. Many horses love hands-on Reiki. They will stand

FULL-BODY HANDS-ON TREATMENT

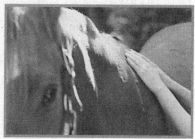

1. The shoulder is a good place to start a hands-on treatment.

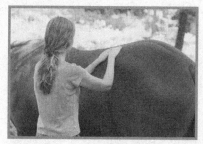

2. Work your way down the spine.

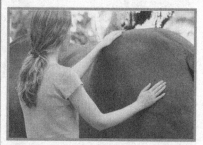

3. Place one hand on the point of the hip, the other on the buttock.

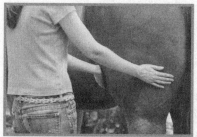

4. Place one hand on the stifle, the other on the thigh.

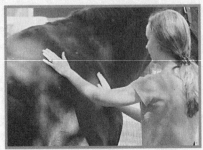

Taller horses may find treatment more comfortable with your hands placed farther apart.

still, grazing or even dozing, as you move around, changing hand positions and moving from side to side during the treatment.

Your horse's shoulder is a good place to start a hands-on treatment (picture 1 on page 105). Most horses feel comfortable when being touched on their shoulders, so it's a great position for them to get used to the feel of hands-on Reiki. Rest your hands lightly, without pressure, on your horse. If this position is not comfortable, your horse will move away from your hands. Don't follow him if he moves; remember, you can offer Reiki from a distance if this is more comfortable for him.

Continue to gently rest your hands on your horse (or hold them a few inches off the skin, if he prefers that) and begin working your way down one side of the spine, shoulder to hip.

Alternate sides as you go, placing both hands on one side of the spine then the other (picture 2 on page 105).

On the hind end, we recommend two basic positions. For the first, place one hand on the point of the hip and the other on the buttock muscle (picture 3 on page 105). For the second, place one hand on the stifle and the other on the buttock. Thus, the back, hip and stifle areas are covered (picture 4 on page 105). Often, when horses have health problems lower down the leg, they prefer you to work from up here; the Reiki goes where it needs to go, and can often feel too intense when given directly over an injury. Your horse will let you know what's comfortable to him.

If you only have time for a 30-minute treatment, try a modified position where your hands

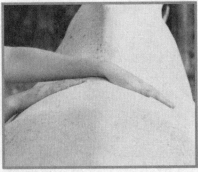

This position, with your hands on both sides of the spine, works well for a pony or small horse.

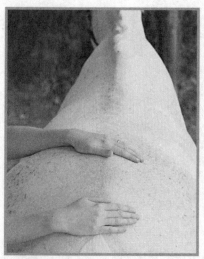

Rather than doing two positions on each hind leg, put your hands over the spine to treat both hind legs at the same time.

the dock. In addition, if your pony or horse isn't comfortable receiving Reiki directly on his legs, this position is usually very acceptable.

TREATING YOUR HORSE'S LEGS

When you've finished treating a horse's body, hands-on treatment of the legs is a nice, optional add-on. Or, if you don't have time to give a complete treatment and your horse has a specific leg injury, you can do a shorter treatment focusing only on the affected leg.

are wider apart. The wider position covers more area, faster. This position also works well for taller horses.

Another time-saving position is to work both sides of the spine at the same time (bottom right picture on page 106). This position is also good for a pony or small horse. Work from shoulder to hip, as with a bigger horse.

To treat both hind legs at the same time (instead of doing each hind leg separately), just put your hands over the spine (see picture above). Often problems in the hind legs respond energetically to this hand position, with one hand over the croup, the other at

When treating a horse's legs, you should always squat nearby, and to the side. Don't put yourself directly in front of or behind the horse. Also, don't sit on the ground, kneel or sit on a stool: If your horse shifts, you want to be able to move away quickly and avoid getting caught underfoot. For extremely nervous horses, or horses that move around a lot or kick, don't try to treat the legs directly.

Start with the front legs (pictures 1–4 on page 108) and then move to the hind legs (pictures 5–8 on page 108). For both front and back legs, start at the body and work down to the hoof, focusing on the joints. If your horse

HANDS-ON TREATMENT OF LEGS

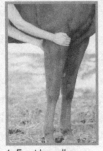
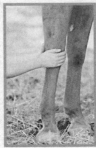
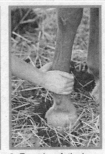
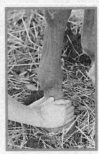

1. Front leg: elbow joint   2. Front leg: knee   3. Front leg: fetlock joint   4. Front leg: the hoof

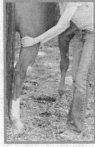
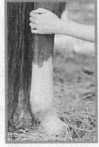
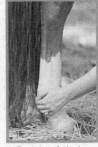
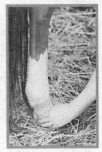

5. Back leg: stifle joint and thigh   6. Back leg: the hock   7. Back leg: fetlock joint   8. Back leg: the hoof

has a specific injury that's not on the joints, you can try treating it directly, if your horse is comfortable with it. However, since joints are little energy centers in your horse's body, they're a good place to focus your hands-on Reiki. The specific way you cover the joints depends on what is comfortable for you and for your horse. You may place your hands around the joint, on the front and back, or on the sides. Experiment to see what works best.

chapter 11

Reiki for Small Animals

SMALL ANIMALS, SUCH AS rabbits, guinea pigs, mice, rats, ferrets, frogs, snakes and lizards, are often comfortable being picked up and held by humans. But being held for love and petting and being held for Reiki are very different things. When Reiki begins flowing from your hands, it can feel too intense for these little creatures, and they may become uncomfortable or feel coerced into the treatment.

Once they sense you are "pushing" the treatment, they won't want to accept Reiki and will try to get away from you. This is why it's especially important to always start treatment from a distance when working with these precious little ones. Whether you leave them in their hutch, cage or aquarium, or put them onto your lap or near you on the floor or couch, always start by asking their permission, letting them know that they need only take the energy they want, and assuring them that you won't force things: this treatment will be their choice and on their terms. Then while resting your hands on your lap, just ask Reiki to start flowing.

They may approach you and crawl into your lap or under your hands. They may turn their bodies around under your hands periodically during the treatment to receive direct contact Reiki for the areas

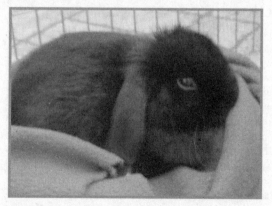

that feel the best for them. They may move away, crawl into their bed and go to sleep for the duration of the treatment. If they're in their cage or aquarium, they'll probably come forward to the place closest to where you're sitting and fall asleep.

Whichever way they choose to receive the treatment is the right way for them. Watch for signs of acceptance in their relaxed behavior: little sighs, falling asleep, or simply becoming very still and settled but not taking their eyes off you. Remember that just because they are small doesn't mean they take less energy or shorter treatments: be ready to spend an average of 30 to 60 minutes and feel a lot of Reiki flowing, even if you're treating the tiniest mouse!

If you have more than one small animal in your household, Reiki can be offered to each animal individually or to all of them together. Group treatment is very effective and can be convenient if you don't have time to offer separate treatments. Sometimes the animals will decide who goes first and take turns receiving their treatments. Sometimes they'll cluster around you as you give the treatment, and you may end up with each hand on a different animal, or an animal under one hand and the others clustered nearby absorbing the energy.

You'll know the treatment is ending when your animal comes

MELVIN AND MONICA

Melvin and Monica were beautiful, black-and-white, long-haired, guinea pigs, about four months old, who had been surrendered to the shelter. They were kept in separate cages because Melvin had not been neutered, but they interacted constantly, often standing up with their paws against the cage looking at each other and conversing. It was clear that they really loved each other and would like to stay together when they went to a new home. Since this would be much more likely to happen if they could be in the same cage, the decision was made to neuter Melvin.

Before I sent him Reiki for the surgery the next day, I told Melvin why he was having the surgery. As I explained to him that he would be able to be with Monica afterward, he began jumping up in the air over and over, doing little pirouettes in mid-air. I'd never seen that behavior from him before and felt he was reacting to the news that he and Monica could be together. When I sat next to his cage, put my hands in my lap, and offered him Reiki for the surgery, he looked at me for a moment and then lay down, flat out on the floor of his cage, closed his eyes, and dozed for about 20 minutes. When he got up, he scampered over to the side of his cage near Monica and began squeaking to her in a very animated way. The surgery went well the next day, he recovered quickly, and the two guinea pigs were overjoyed when they were finally allowed to live together. —*Elizabeth*

A NEW TURTLE FRIEND

One day I arrived to pick up my daughter from summer camp and learned that they had planned an extra half hour of activities that day and so I was early. I wandered around the facility while I waited until I noticed an enclosure with a large turtle in it. I sat down by the enclosure to observe the turtle, who was resting on the far side of the enclosure. After a few minutes I decided to offer him Reiki while I waited. I explained what I was going to do and asked the turtle to take only the energy he wished to receive. Then I put my hands down on my lap and let the energy flow to him. After about ten minutes the turtle began to move over toward me. He came about midway across the enclosure and stopped for a minute or two. Finally he came over into the corner nearest me and positioned himself right under my hands, which by then I was holding over him at lap level with the palms facing down toward him. He rested there peacefully until my daughter arrived, and it was time to end the treatment. —*Elizabeth*

out of his quiet, relaxed state and becomes involved in another activity. If he offers you a gesture of gratitude, this is another sign that he's finished with the treatment. At about the same time, you'll usually notice a decrease in the level of energy flowing through your hands and you may find that your attention is beginning to turn to other matters. At the end of the treatment, always thank Reiki for the healing it has brought about and the animal for his participation.

Fish and water-dwelling creatures   Reiki is a wonderful healing modality for fish, eels, tadpoles, sea urchins, anemones and other water-dwelling creatures. Fish and other water-dwellers are extremely delicate and sensitive

to all things, and Reiki is a gentle, effective way to bring healing to them. The water environment in which fish live is an exquisite receptor and transmitter of energy. Much research has been done over the last century in the fields of physics and chemistry to show that water absorbs energy and retains the memory and properties of the energy that's absorbed by it. More recently, Dr. Masaru Emoto has shown that the energy of human thoughts, words and feelings is absorbed by water and results in changes in its basic structure.

The watery environment in which companion fish live in a household absorbs the energies around it, and fish are continually passing this water through their bodies by way of their gills. Offering Reiki to your fish provides them with healing on all levels of their being and, in addition, has the ability to clear their water environment of any energetic influences that may not be healthy for them. Fish, especially goldfish, can be attuned to the people in their environment, so sending Reiki to yourself and your situation with your fish can be a very effective way to bring healing to them. Like other animals, fish can become stressed by tensions and emotions in the household and can benefit greatly from a mental and emotional healing, if you have Level 2 Reiki.

Because fish are so sensitive, offering Reiki to them at a little bit of a distance is generally the best idea. When we give treatments to fish, we follow the same principles that we use for treating other animals. We explain what Reiki is to the fish and ask them to take only as much Reiki as they wish to receive. We tell them they are in control of the treatment and can draw the amount of energy they want to themselves. Then we rest our hands at a short distance from the tank or aquarium and allow the energy to flow to the fish.

All of the indicators of acceptance of Reiki that you see with other animals also occur with fish. They may at first be wary of the energy and may move away from your hands, but eventually they may come up to the side of the aquarium to be closer to the

KI KOI

I was once asked to heal a tiny koi, who was sick and hadn't eaten for some time; because of the fish's small size and fragility, her person was worried that she wouldn't recover. When I first saw her, she was so ill, she was laying at a 45-degree angle at the bottom of the bowl. I placed my hands near the container, about six inches away, and began to offer Reiki.

For such a tiny fish, she took an incredible amount of energy! After about 30 minutes of treatment, I felt the energy dissipate. I noticed she seemed to be breathing with less difficulty, but she still wasn't swimming, or even upright. The next day, her person emailed me to let me know that within an hour of the treatment, she ate three worms and was now, a day later, swimming around energetically again. She decided to name her Ki Koi because of her affinity and response to Reiki energy. She's still doing great, and growing bigger every day! —*Kathleen*

energy. If this occurs, you may want to move your hands closer to the tank. Because fish and their water environment are so intertwined, placing your hands on the tank initially can be too intense for fish; they'll feel the energy very strongly when your hands are on the tank, and the intensity of the feeling may alarm them if they haven't had a chance to become accustomed to it at a distance. Since they're so extremely sensitive, fish and other water-dwellers can respond very quickly to Reiki healing, as the Ki Koi story on page 112 illustrates.

Reptiles and amphibians Like other animals, reptiles and amphibians are drawn to Reiki's gentle healing. In the wild, many reptiles and amphibians depend on the energy and heat of the sun for their physical needs as well as their needs on intangible emotional and spiritual levels. In captivity, even with the best artificial lighting available, they're missing some of the benefits of the sun and a connection to the natural world.

In offering Reiki to reptiles and amphibians, it's ideal if the animal is free to move around and choose whether to come to your hands or remain at a dis-tance. If this is not possible, you can sit at a small distance just outside the animal's enclosure and offer Reiki to him from there. As with other animals, explaining to him what you're doing and asking him to take only the amount of energy he wants will greatly increase the likelihood that he'll embrace a treatment.

Reiki can provide some of what's missing in captive, indoor life with its ability to nurture and heal on both physical and emotional levels. Like other animals, reptiles and amphibians can become stressed by tension and emotional turmoil in the household and can benefit greatly from a mental and emotional healing, if you have Level 2 Reiki.

The treatment will begin when you allow the Reiki energy to flow from your hands. As with other animals, reptiles and amphibians may take some time to assess the new energy and may come closer to you and go away again while they do so. Eventually they'll often end up peacefully dozing nearby, enjoying the new sensation and its many benefits. Some snakes will even come up and curl in your hands to be close to the Reiki energy.

GODIVA'S REMARKABLE RECOVERY

Even traumatized animals respond well to Reiki when given control over the treatment. When first adopted by my sister, Godiva was an extremely withdrawn guinea pig who had been kept in a dark closet and roughly handled by a child. She went inside her house whenever she saw a person and, unlike most guinea pigs, moved very little, never played and barely made any vocalizations.

My sister was concerned that she perhaps had some kind of brain damage because she was so unresponsive. She huddled out of my sight in her house as I introduced myself to her and began to offer her Reiki from just outside the cage. I reassured her that I wouldn't force any kind of contact with her and that she need only accept the healing energy if she wanted it. I mentally let her know she was in a safe place now.

As soon as I began the treatment, she peeked her head outside her house, made eye contact, rested her head on her paws, and made a little sigh. I felt the flow of Reiki very strongly. She remained in that position, watching me, and after half an hour, I felt the flow of energy dissipate and ended the treatment. I thanked Reiki and then thanked Godiva for her willingness to heal.

As I sat down on a couch nearby to discuss the treatment, Godiva suddenly came out of her house, put her front legs on the bars of the cage nearest to me, and began to squeak loudly over and over. My sister exclaimed in amazement that she had only made that noise once or twice when she was getting fed her favorite food: fresh lettuce. It was a clear, "Thanks for the Reiki!"

With frequent Reiki treatments, in combination with my sister's patient care, a new fresh food regimen, and regular doses of fresh air and sunlight, Godiva made an amazing recovery. She grew to love the touch of human hands, even purring and squeaking when scratched.

Her healing progress was tested most recently when a large production crew moved into my sister's home for a couple of days to film an episode of HGTV's *Design Remix*. Despite all the unfamiliar people, equipment and noise, Godiva remained unfazed. At the end of the shoot, one of the crew remarked to my sister, "You have the most outgoing and friendly guinea pig I've ever seen!" What amazing progress this little girl has made. Thank you, Reiki. —*Kathleen*

■ Overview of the treatment

The approach Always ask permission first, letting the animal know that he need only take the energy he wants, and let him come to you.

Treating from a distance Begin your treatment at a distance. Reiki will be effective for your small animal friend even if you offer Reiki from outside the cage. The most important factors are your intention and the animal's acceptance, not the proximity of your hands to his body.

Basic body positions Sit near your animal and let him come and investigate your hands. If he crawls into your hands or your lap, that's a sure sign that he wants hands-on Reiki. Just put your hands directly on his body, or rest them several inches away—whatever seems most comfortable to your animal. Allow him to move around the treatment space and come close to or move away from your hands as he chooses.

Finishing the treatment Remember to thank Reiki for the healing it has brought and to thank your animal for his participation. You may want to spend a few minutes with him for affection, scratches and pats at the end of the treatment.

(see Chapters 4 and 5 for further information)

▬ Basic treatment

Some animals have a preference for treatment from a distance, especially when they first experience Reiki. After you ask permission to begin the treatment, your animal may come over to investigate your hands, as Godiva does in picture 1 below. In this way she shows that she is accepting the energy, and even more, that she is curious about it.

If your animal cannot move about freely without a cage, it's best to treat her from outside her cage, with your arms lowered and your palms facing up. Holding your hands against the cage and pointing them toward your animal may be experienced as coercive and is not a good idea unless your animal comes forward, inviting you to place your hands against the cage.

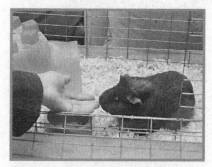
1. Godiva accepts the Reiki treatment.

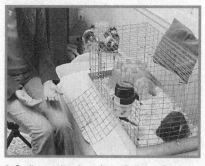
2. Godiva settles down for a "Reiki nap."

Your animal may then move away and settle down for a "Reiki nap" (see picture 2 on page 115). Rather than try to put your hands directly on her, rest your hands on your lap, allowing your animal to relax and take Reiki from a distance.

After resting, dozing or sleeping for a while, your animal may get up and drink some water, get involved in another activity, or offer a gesture of gratitude. This is often a sign that the treatment is over. Take a few moments to thank your animal for her acceptance of the healing energy.

Reiki treatments may be both hands-on and from a distance, as Ted the toad's story exemplifies. Ted, who came to BrightHaven animal sanctuary with no back legs from the knees down and unable to eat on his own, doesn't mind being held. But even in this case, Kathleen does not assume that he wants his Reiki treatment to be hands-on. She says hello to Ted and asks his permission to begin the treatment (picture 1 below). She then finds a comfortable place for Ted to be during the treatment.

By placing her hands at some distance from Ted, she ensures he's free to choose whether to take the treatment or not (picture 2 below). As the Reiki begins flowing, Ted shows that he appreciates the energy by hopping closer to Kathleen's right hand and settling down, becoming completely still and relaxed. In addition, because Ted's free to hop away, he's able to determine how long the treatment will last.

After lots of loving care and a warm, safe home environment, Ted is now able to eat on his own, and actually gets around

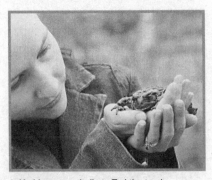

1. Kathleen says hello to Ted the toad.

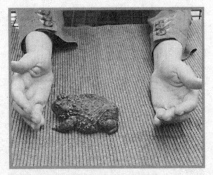

2. Ted basks in his Reiki treatment.

pretty well, even without part of his back legs. In fact, Ted doesn't like to sit still, so it was amazing to everyone how motionless and relaxed he remained for his entire Reiki treatment!

chapter 12

Reiki for Farm Animals

FARM ANIMALS SUCH AS COWS, PIGS, goats and chickens are usually not used to getting much TLC from humans. If your farm animals are rescues from a factory or commercial farm, they may have survived abuse at the hands of humans, and may not wish close contact, or may show fear when approached. This is why Reiki is an ideal therapy to help them recover. With Reiki, you can sit outside their pen, ask permission, letting them know that they need only take the energy they want, and just let the Reiki begin flowing. Even if they don't trust most people and have less than positive memories of human contact, when they sense the healing energy coming from you, without coercion, they'll become interested in what you have to offer.

If you sit quietly and do not force eye contact, they may come over to you and smell your hands through the fence or simply watch you very seriously. In time, with repeated treatments, you can rebuild the trust that was lost and help the animal heal from his past. Not only will Reiki give

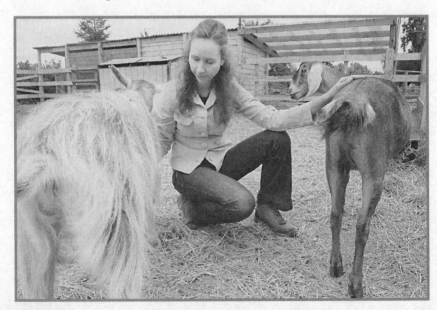

HARLEY THE GENTLE GIANT

Harley came to live at BrightHaven animal sanctuary in 2002, barely rescued from becoming someone's pork product. A young pig when he arrived, Harley had lots of energy (and especially enjoyed digging and rooting), a quality that proved challenging for the staff and volunteers. But his gentle nature continued to grow, as did his size.

Now around 800 pounds, Harley is a favorite among visitors to BrightHaven; he loves attention, scratches and hugs. The first time I tried Reiki with Harley, I was rather intimidated because of his size. I spoke to him from across his field (safely from outside the fence) and asked him if he'd like some Reiki. Then I settled in next to the fence line and began sending the energy.

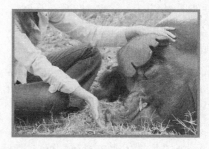

Harley immediately got up from the place where he was napping, walked purposefully across the field, stuck his nose through the fence and pushed at my hands with his snout. After some excited oinking, he turned around and lay down, pushing his hind legs against the fence where I sat. It was obvious that he wanted some hands-on Reiki. As soon as I put my hands on his legs, he stretched his head down to the ground and fell asleep. His little corkscrew of a tail became so relaxed, it straightened all the way out!

When I finished, I thanked Harley, and as I walked away, he lifted his head and watched me go. Then he promptly got up and walked into his house for a nap. In speaking to Gail about the treatment, I learned some interesting details about Harley's physical health. For the last year or so, he's had some difficulty and discomfort with his hind end. It's a condition caused in part by his heavy weight, and helped a great deal by homeopathic remedies. It amazed me that Harley was able to understand so quickly what Reiki was, and exactly the area he needed to focus on. Now when Harley sees me coming, he knows what I'm there for and lays down for a relaxing treatment. —*Kathleen*

such animals the emotional healing that is needed, but your role as the "provider" of Reiki will help them form new, positive memories of contact with humans.

If you have farm animals with whom you have a close relationship, perhaps even having delivered them into this world yourself, Reiki will not only heal them in the ways they need most, but also deepen your relationship with them in a rich and rewarding way. When they realize you have healing energy to

DOROTHY THE GOAT

BrightHaven animal sanctuary saved Dorothy from euthanasia at the pound in 2001. She was being treated for mastitis there and was rescued by a vet tech at the hospital who was asked to euthanize her. She arrived extremely malnourished, with an injury to her front right leg. Over time, with good food, love and homeopathy, her weight and strength returned, along with her sparkling and stubborn personality. Wonderfully, the vet tech who rescued her became a BrightHaven volunteer.

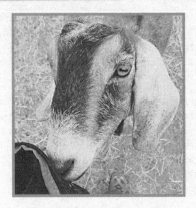

Interestingly, Dorothy seems to seek out Reiki for her old leg injury, even though she has shown no symptoms for some time. When receiving Reiki treatments, Dorothy likes to spend part of the time receiving Reiki hands-on to her front right leg, but also likes to walk away and receive part of the treatment from a distance. Once she realizes that she isn't being coerced to participate and that I'm letting her choose how to receive her treatment, she usually comes right back to my hands, lowering her head and relaxing as I place my hands over her leg. Dorothy gets jealous when she thinks her goat buddy, Paloma, might be trying to share in the hands-on part of the treatment. There's been some head butting to settle things. She seems happy to share Reiki with Paloma, though, as long as it's from a distance. —*Kathleen*

offer them, they'll begin to come to you when they need healing. In many cases, they'll tell you exactly where they need Reiki by putting specific parts of their body directly into your hands and resting quietly for the duration of the treatment.

The wonderful gift you'll receive when treating farm animals with Reiki is that in experiencing the healing possibilities and warm responses from these animals, you'll get a glimpse into their world. You'll truly be able to appreciate the depth of their emotions and the fullness of their lives in a way that you may have otherwise overlooked.

■ Overview of the treatment

The approach　Always ask permission, letting the animal know that he need only take the energy he wants, before you begin. Depending on your comfort level and that of the animal you're working with, you may choose to work from outside the enclosure.

Treating from a distance Like most animals, farm animals appreciate it if you begin the treatment from a distance and allow them to approach if they want hands-on treatment.

Basic body positions For larger animals, start on the shoulders and work towards the hind end, alternating sides. For smaller animals, just choose a position with one or both hands on the body (see Poodle the chicken's treatment on page 131). In either case, don't shift positions if it disturbs the relaxed state of the

HANDS-ON REIKI TREATMENT

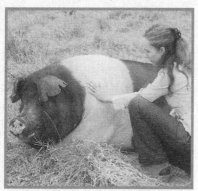
1. Harley agrees to a Reiki treatment.

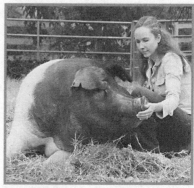
2. Harley continues to explore the source of the Reiki energy.

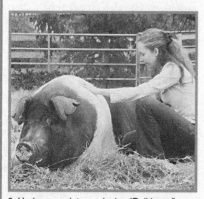
3. Harley goes into a relaxing "Reiki nap."

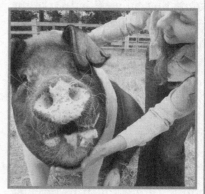
4. Harley wakes up: treatment is over.

animal. Sometimes animals, especially small animals, prefer only one hand on them. Start with one hand and add the other if the animal seems comfortable with it.

Extra positions You may choose to do hand positions on the head and legs, if the animal offers you these parts for treatment.

Finishing the treatment Thank the animal for his participation. You can spend a few moments of TLC time, if the animal enjoys it.

(see Chapters 4 and 5 for further information)

▰ Basic treatment

Some farm animals are very affectionate and close with humans and may love hands-on Reiki. However, it is best to always begin a treatment by asking permission and letting the animal know that he need only take the energy he wants. Carefully watch his body language for permission. As Reiki begins flowing, your animal may investigate your hands, feeling the energy. You will see signs of relaxation if your animal agrees to the treatment. Once you receive this permission, you can settle into a comfortable position from which to treat. Be open to your animal settling quietly under your hands, or moving to and from your hands throughout the treatment. The most important thing is that your animal has the freedom to receive the treatment in the ways that are most comfortable for him.

Harley the pig's treatment on page 121 is a great example of what a typical Reiki treatment will look like for an animal that chooses to settle quietly for the duration of the treatment. Harley is a very affectionate pig who loves hands-on Reiki. Still, Kathleen always begins by asking permission, letting him know that he need only take the energy he wants, and carefully watches his body language for permission. He investigates Kathleen's hands as the Reiki begins flowing. He stays very relaxed, saying yes to Reiki, so she gets into a comfortable position for the treatment's duration (picture 1 on page 121).

In picture 2 on page 121, Harley remains very aware and engaged during the first part of the treatment, even leaning into Kathleen's hands. He continually wants to smell her palms, as if to ask, "What's in there?" After 10 to 15 minutes, Harley settles in for his "Reiki nap" (picture 3 on

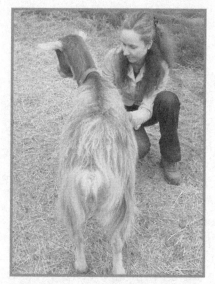
1. Dorothy the goat receives treatment on her front leg.

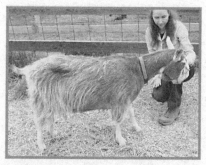
2. Dorothy nudges Kathleen's hand during the treatment.

page 121). It's often during this quiet time that the most powerful healing can occur.

During the treatment, Harley yawns several times, another way that he's showing that he's open and accepting of the healing being offered. The treatment is over when he gets up from his nap (picture 4 on page 121). When thanked, Harley responds with a loud chorus of joyful oinks as he returns thanks to Kathleen for the treatment.

Though some farm animals like Harley may remain in the same spot while receiving Reiki, others tend to move around throughout the treatment. In Dorothy the goat's case, as soon as Kathleen asks permission and begins to offer the energy, Dorothy comes right over and presents her front right leg, which has an old injury (picture 1 on this page).

Dorothy moves away, and then comes back to Kathleen's hands: this is normal behavior for animals, and Kathleen just backs up to the fence, giving Dorothy even more space than she has asked for. As soon as Dorothy realizes Kathleen isn't following her, she returns to Kathleen and nudges her hands (picture 2 on this page). This shows that Dorothy accepts the treatment, and appreciates that Kathleen allowed her to choose how to receive the energy.

chapter 13

Reiki for Birds

BIRDS ARE VERY INTELLIGENT AND PLAYFUL creatures and often have strong personalities, likes and dislikes. They are highly emotional beings, forming close attachments to their special human and bird companions and sometimes displaying strong feelings of jealousy and rivalry toward other humans or animals in the household. Using Reiki with your bird is a way to maintain his health, to help heal any illnesses or injuries that arise, and to deepen and enhance your bond with each other. It's also a way to heal situations that arise with other people or birds. Connecting with your bird through Reiki will also bring you a deeper understanding of his world and his perspective.

If you're living with a bird who's attached to another person in your household and not particularly fond of you, offering Reiki to the bird and to your relationship with him can be a way of healing it. Using Reiki can also bring harmony to the relationship between your bird and other animals in your home. Reiki can help with stress-related ailments like feather plucking. Reiki can also offer peace and comfort to a bird who may be depressed from losing a friend or mate.

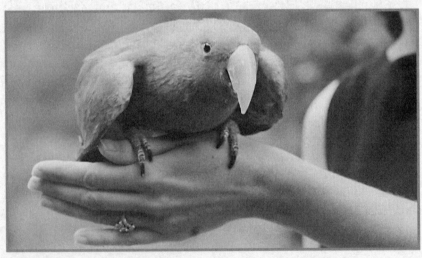

NEW BEGINNINGS

Birds have long lives when they receive good care and sometimes out-live their person. If you have adopted a bird whose previous person passed away, Reiki can help your bird to work through and release his grief so that he can be open to his new relationship with you. When people are no longer able to care for a bird and have to find him a new home, Reiki can bring comfort and healing for the grief and sorrow he may have as a result of the separation. If you have Level 2 Reiki, you can send mental and emotional healing to your bird for any emotional issues he may have as result of things that have happened to him before he came to you.

During a Reiki treatment your bird should be in a place where he feels safe and where the two of you will be undisturbed. Some possibilities are his cage or aviary or a favorite perch in the room with you. The ideal place is one where you can sit or stand comfortably and where your bird can move around freely. If you have more than one bird, you can offer Reiki to both together and let each bird decide whether and how he'll receive the treatment.

Your treatment will be much more successful if you let your bird approach you for Reiki, rather than the other way around. It's best to let go of your expectations for the treatment, and let him determine how things will go.

Before you begin sending Reiki, ask your bird to take only the energy he wants; you want to let him know that he'll be in control of the treatment and that you won't be coercing his participation. To begin the treatment, you can sit or stand at a short distance from him, with your hands lowered at your sides or on your lap, and let the Reiki energy flow to him.

Birds are extremely sensitive creatures, and your bird will feel the energy immediately. Before long you'll usually see signs of interest and acceptance from your bird, such as approaching you to investigate your hands, looking curiously at you, lowering his head, fluffing out his feathers, making contented noises, or settling in for a "Reiki nap." If you're sending Reiki to a relationship or situation in addition to sending it to your bird, you may focus your thoughts on this as you send Reiki to your bird.

It's very common for birds to come and go from your hands, and you should allow them to do so and refrain from following them if they move away. Just as you'll often feel the ebb and flow of the energy in your hands during the treatment, there's an ebb and flow in the way many animals take a treatment. For instance, they may move closer to you and then farther away, or they may settle against your hands and then move away and come back. The pattern may be repeated several times during a treatment.

Birds generally prefer Reiki at a short distance but sometimes enjoy hands-on treatment, especially after they become familiar with Reiki. The choice should always be theirs. If your bird chooses to take the treatment from a distance, he may settle quietly near you or at a distance and doze or fall asleep. If your bird wants your hands on him, he'll come to you, settle quietly

SUNSHINE'S STORY

Several years ago, my sister Maureen adopted a beautiful cockatiel named Sunshine. She had been living in a dark garage because her people thought she was "too loud and made too much of a mess." The same day Maureen heard of her plight, she drove right over and rescued her. At first, due to her past, Sunshine was very fearful of people.

Maureen's boyfriend Mike, a Reiki practitioner, began to offer Sunshine Reiki treatments to help her overcome her fear. Over time, with all the light, love, Reiki and attention showered upon her in her new home, Sunshine really "came out of her shell." Her favorite activity was to take a bath in a small bowl of water, and she loved being scratched on the bright orange circle on her cheek. She had the full run of the apartment, using her beak to help her climb the sides of the furniture. Mike began to spend more time with her, even taking her home to live with him, and they developed a deep bond; he began referring to her affectionately as "Farnsworth."

Maureen and Mike loved to play peek-a-boo with her in the evenings. Each evening, they'd let her out of her cage and she'd run and hide behind the cage. She'd gradually peek her head around the corner, and when they saw her, they'd exclaim, "Peek a boo!" She'd duck her head and run behind the cage, gradually peeking out her head again from the other side. This game would go on for several minutes each evening, with her making cute cooing noises as they played.

under your hands, and often nap for the entire session. Your bird may walk or fly over to you and place his head or body directly into your hands, or he may perch nearby on your shoulder for a nap to be near the Reiki energy. If your bird's wings are clipped, you may need to assist him in coming closer to you for Reiki, if you get the impression that this is what he wants to do.

You will know the treatment is ending when your bird comes out of his quiet, relaxed state and becomes involved in another activity, such as singing, playing, whistling, eating or drinking. If your bird offers you a gesture of gratitude, this is another sign that he's finished with the treatment. When birds have had enough Reiki, they often thank you with a kiss, a nuzzle or a push of their beak, or make happy sounds before moving away from you and returning to other matters. At about the same time you'll usually notice a

---

In time Sunshine fell in love with Mike, even thinking he was her mate. Because she was so happy and comfortable, Sunshine loved to lay eggs and would often sit on the floor of her cage, or just outside on a blanket my sister provided for her. When I visited, I'd occasionally spend some time sitting nearby Sunshine and offering her Reiki. She always showed the same behavior during treatments: she'd plump up her feathers, close her eyes and fall asleep.

One night, Mike came home late and noticed that Sunshine was sitting in the open door of her cage, swaying back and forth and definitely not looking right. He became very concerned and took her on his finger over to the bed. He lay down and put her on his stomach. She wasn't moving at all, which was very uncharacteristic. He gently put his hand over her body so that just her head peeked out, and offered her Reiki for about ten minutes. Suddenly, she got a great burst of energy and playfulness, running up his shirt to his chest, where she began biting his necklace and earrings, behavior she regularly showed as a form of affection for Mike. It was as if she were thanking him for the Reiki treatment. He felt relieved that she seemed so much better, and so put her back into her cage for the night.

That night, Sunshine passed away, from causes unknown to the veterinarian: perhaps she had complications due to her egg laying, or perhaps she had injured herself flying. Her loss was quite a shock to Maureen and Mike, who loved her dearly, but they both were comforted to know that Reiki helped make her last evening—and indeed her life—more comfortable. —*Kathleen*

A COCKATIEL'S GIFT OF LOVE

Pamela is the head of a bird sanctuary on the east coast. She contacted me when her favorite bird Lenore, a cockatiel, was at the end of her life and getting close to making her transition. Lenore was the first bird Pamela rescued and the reason she started the sanctuary 12 years before. She was the matriarch of the large flock of birds and was deferred to in most circumstances by all the birds. Pamela and Lenore had a close connection and, while Lenore had relationships with the other birds and took her status with them seriously, she preferred Pamela's company to that of any of the birds.

Pamela wanted to do everything she could to repay Lenore for all she had taught her about birds and their care, and to make her last days and her passing as comfortable and easy as possible. She asked me to send her a series of four distant Reiki treatments to help her in her transition. In each of the treatments I received a strong wave of grief that lasted for several minutes, sometimes bringing tears to my eyes or even leaving me sobbing, as Lenore progressively let out her sadness at having to leave her beloved person. Lenore also sent a strong sense of her pride in having started the sanctuary and in being Pamela's teacher about the ways of birds. Less than a week later, Lenore made her transition peacefully at home. —*Elizabeth*

decrease in the level of energy flowing through your hands.

Reiki always goes where it's needed, so if your bird is comfortable with one hand position throughout the treatment, you can listen to him and trust that he'll get exactly the amount of Reiki that he needs from this one position. As you become familiar with Reiki, your bird's behavior will guide you in learning how to give the right treatment. And as your experience with Reiki grows, your intuition about your bird's health and preferences, as well as your understanding of his mental and emotional state, will deepen.

■ Overview of the treatment

The approach Ask your bird for permission before you begin. Allow your bird to approach you, not the other way around. Be sensitive to his body language to see if he's open to receiving the energy. He should become engaged and, eventually, relaxed.

Treating from a distance Stand or sit near the perch or cage where your bird feels most comfortable. Watch your bird for signs of relaxation and interest. Each bird will take Reiki in his own unique way, and each treatment of the same bird may be different; therefore, it's important to begin each treatment from a distance, even if you know your bird well and treat him with Reiki regularly. By beginning at a distance, you'll give him the freedom to show you how he wants to receive Reiki in each new treatment.

Basic hand positions Most birds prefer to receive Reiki from a short distance, so avoid hands-on Reiki with your bird unless he asks for it. If your bird does want hands-on Reiki, find a position on his body that he's comfortable with and allow him to reposition himself as he wishes.

Finishing the treatment When your bird wakes up or "comes out" of his relaxed state and resumes his normal activities, this is a sign the treatment is finished. Spend a few moments thanking your bird for his participation in the treatment.

(see Chapters 4 and 5 for further information)

▬ Treatment from a short distance

Stand near your bird, ask permission, letting him know he need only take the energy he wants,

and begin to offer Reiki energy. He'll probably come over close to you, showing immediate interest in the energy.

Another option is to sit near your bird and place your hands in a comfortable position. Watch your bird for signs that he's enjoying the energy, such as relaxation or eye contact.

A Reiki treatment for an adolescent cockatoo named Birdie shows how Reiki often brings about healing in surprising ways. Birdie was boarding at a pet shop where Elizabeth offered Reiki with her daughter Laura. The first day he arrived, Birdie screamed

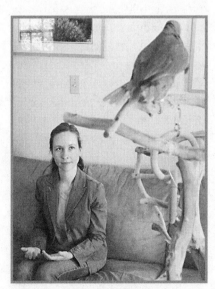

You can sit (or stand) next to your bird when giving Reiki from a short distance.

non-stop. The staff was frantic and felt they couldn't endure the racket for the month they had agreed to board him. They asked Elizabeth and Laura to help. Elizabeth stood near the cage, hands lowered by her sides in an offering position, and asked Birdie's permission to give a treatment. Within minutes Birdie became absolutely quiet, gradually moving closer to Elizabeth until finally he was pressed against the side of the cage, relaxed, with his head hanging low, looking comically blissful.

After the treatment, he was much quieter, shrieking only a few times. Just before Elizabeth left, one of the staff suddenly had the idea of putting Birdie's cage in the window, where he could see the people outside as well as the activity in the shop. Birdie was moved and he never shrieked again, behaving perfectly for the rest of the month.

▬ Hands-on treatment

Take the time to say hello to your bird and ask permission before you start, letting him know he need only take the energy he wants. If your bird enjoys being held, find the most comfortable way for him to be with you. Most birds won't want your hands directly over their backs during a treatment, although there are exceptions. Follow your bird's wishes by observing his body language to determine the best way to give the treatment.

Once you've found a comfortable position, it's possible to do the whole treatment from this

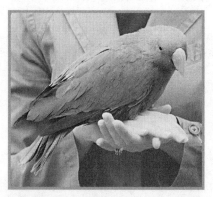

1. Picasso finds a comfortable perch.

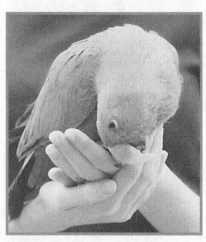

2. A playful Picasso enjoys his Reiki treatment.

position without disturbing your bird's relaxation. Picasso, an Eclectic parrot, had trouble perching on the side of Kathleen's hand, so she placed her hand flat with the other hand underneath for added stability (see picture 1 on page 130). Once he felt comfortable, he was able to relax and enjoy the treatment.

Birds can often become very happy and energetic as well as curious about your hands during the treatment. Watch your bird for signs that he's enjoying the energy such as head bobbing, making happy noises, yawning or even sleeping. In picture 2 on page 130, Picasso is clearly enjoying himself.

Sometimes, birds you think would not accept hands-on treatment may surprise you. Poodle, a silky chicken with a hairstyle like a fancy dog and a personality like a cat, is the most pampered bird at BrightHaven. She demands to be fed from her own separate bowl at a distance from the other birds. She loves being petted and held, responding just as a cat would to petting and attention.

On Kathleen's first visit with Poodle, she squatted down to be lower and closer to "bird" level,

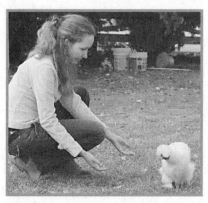

1. Poodle comes over to greet Kathleen.

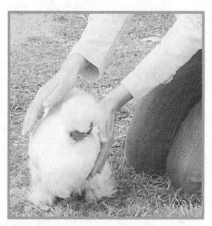

2. Poodle appreciates hands-on Reiki, becoming very relaxed and still during treatment.

and first just said hello to Poodle and all the other birds there. Kathleen then introduced herself and asked permission to begin giving Reiki. As she began offering the energy, she left her focus open to anyone in the bird pasture who wanted Reiki.

Poodle showed immediate interest in the energy, moving

PD THE PARROT

PD is a six-year-old Amazon parrot, probably a Yellow head mix. He has been with his human family since he was three months old. He's confident, athletic and very bonded to and protective of his special human companion, Emily. Along with Emily, he shares his home with a dad, two children, three dogs, a kitten, a turtle and two parakeets. The other animals know PD's in charge! Although a well-mannered guy, he can get lonely and chew his feet if Emily isn't around to spend time with him every day. PD doesn't always take to strangers, so Emily was very pleased at his ability to relax and interact with me when I came to offer Reiki. —*Kathleen*

close to Kathleen and looking at her hands (picture 1 on page 131). Because of previous experience doing Reiki with chickens, Kathleen assumed Poodle would want her treatment from a short distance but Poodle was open to hands-on Reiki. Poodle remained quiet and peaceful for the entire treatment (picture 2 on page 131). When Poodle had enough Reiki, she simply walked away from Kathleen's hands. Kathleen thanked her new friend and gave Poodle a few scratches under the chin.

chapter 14

Reiki for Senior and Special-Needs Animals

▬ Senior animals

As our animals grow older, they become more fragile, sometimes losing their sight or hearing, and have more difficulty moving around. Reiki is a great way to reduce your animal's symptoms and provide comfort and relief to him for the symptoms he does develop. Using Reiki regularly with your aging animal will keep you in touch with how he's feeling and provide moments of priceless intimacy as he grows older.

When offering Reiki to your senior animal, begin by asking him to take only the amount of Reiki that he wants and assuring him that he'll be in control of the treatment. As in all situations, hands-on Reiki is appropriate only when your animal asks for it. Senior animals are often more sensitive to many things, including energy, than they were earlier in their lives, and Reiki can feel very intense to them at first. Beginning the treatment at a distance and allowing your animal to

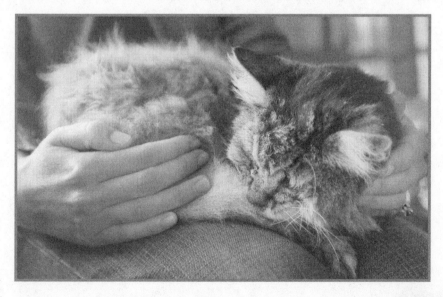

come to you if he wants your hands on him will assure him the most comfortable and effective treatment.

Even when your animal seeks out hands-on Reiki, Reiki can sometimes feel too intense when given directly to an area affected by illness or injury. Using hand positions at a slight distance from the affected area is often the best choice, especially if your animal shows signs of discomfort. For instance, if your animal seems to find Reiki too intense with your hands directly on his arthritic joint, placing your hands on the joint above it can provide comfort and relief from pain. Some animals will prefer your hands directly on the affected area and may position it into your hands. An animal's preferences can change from one treatment to the next, so remember to let your animal be your guide in how to approach each treatment.

▬ Disabled animals/ animals with chronic illness

If your animal is disabled or living with a chronic illness, Reiki can help relieve discomfort and distress and sometimes can even help slow the progression of his condition. A Reiki treatment is a

JOEY: GUARDIAN AND PROTECTOR OF BRIGHTHAVEN

Joey is a giant spirit in a small body: tough as nails and a ball of spunk! Joey came to BrightHaven animal sanctuary after an unfortunate car accident left him without the use of his hind legs; however, the custom canine wheelchair gets him around the house just fine. Most visitors will meet Joey as soon as they arrive; the sound of wheels rolling and "watchdog" barking will follow you as you enter the house. Once he's sure you're "OK," he'll leave you and resume his place at Gail's side.

Joey can be suspicious of strangers, but from the very first time I visited Bright-Haven, he has accepted not only my presence, but also the Reiki I have to offer. Sometimes, he prefers not to be the "focus" of the session, settling at my feet for a Reiki snooze while I'm sitting on a couch treating cats on my lap. Other times, he waits patiently for me to sit down next to him and climbs partially into my lap for the treatment. In most Reiki treatments for Joey, I also focus on mental healing for his anxiety and stress. This is not a quick fix but a long-term project in healing for him. It's a big job to protect all of Bright-Haven's human and animal residents, and Joey takes this job seriously. Regular Reiki treatments help Joey's stress level to be more manageable. —*Kathleen*

wonderful respite for animals living with some form of discomfort or impaired function. When he's having a tough day, a Reiki treatment can help your animal become more centered and comfortable.

A good example of this is Ollie, a 20-year-young Dachshund who, romping around the house in his canine wheelchair, doesn't realize his age. But he's not always so lively. He suffers from recurrent meningitis, and recently began to have a bad episode during a Reiki class Kathleen was giving at BrightHaven animal sanctuary. Fortunately, she was able to treat him with Reiki right then, before the full onset of symptoms, which can include high fever and even seizures. Ollie began taking the energy immediately, and was able to fall asleep for almost 30 minutes. He continued to look uncomfortable for the rest of the day, but by the next day he seemed better.

Ollie did not come down with the disease as he usually did, recovering fully within a few days. And since the treatment, he has been so lively that most mornings he jumps around and barks like a puppy. Now when-

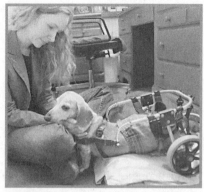

Ollie begins accepting Reiki by investigating Kathleen's hands and then leaning against her lap for the duration of the treatment.

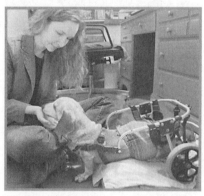

Ollie thanks Kathleen for the treatment by licking her hands, a common way animals show their appreciation for healing energy.

ever Ollie receives Reiki, he continually smells Kathleen's hands, pushing on them with his wet nose, as if to say, "What's in there?"

Sometimes animals begin to resist repeated medical rituals, such as having to swallow lots of pills or enduring the administration of subcutaneous hydration.

In such cases, you can offer Reiki to help the situation. You can also give Reiki to yourself before you give the medicine, focusing on making the process go more easily and smoothly.

Since caring for a disabled animal or one with a chronic illness can be as stressful for you as your animal friend, remember to give yourself Reiki to maintain your own health and to remain centered and balanced so that you can care for your animal in the best way you can.

Establishing a Reiki support network can reduce your stress as you care for your aging, disabled or chronically ill animal. Having a fellow Reiki practitioner send Reiki to you and/or your animal, if you need time off or are feeling overwhelmed, can help keep you from experiencing the burnout that caregivers can feel.

▬ Reiki to the rescues

Rescued animals sometimes come from abusive or neglectful pasts. Through no fault of their own, they can display many behavioral problems that result from emotional damage they have suffered before they came to you. Reiki can reduce and sometimes even eliminate behavioral problems that are emotionally based. You don't need to know the source of their problems, even though you may have a general idea about what they faced in the past. Regardless of your knowledge of the past, Reiki will go straight to the source of their problem and truly heal it, not just take away the symptoms. It can reach deeply into the heart and soul of an animal and is amazing in this way.

During a treatment, you may get an insight or intuition about emotional or spiritual issues concerning your animal. If you have Level 2 Reiki, you can send mental, emotional and spiritual healing to your animal for the challenges he's facing, whether they're mental stress accompanying physical challenges or emotional injuries he may have received in the past. Using Reiki regularly with your animal will help develop your intuition about your animal and the communication between you.

Sometimes a few treatments will bring about dramatic changes; at other times, just as with humans, the healing of emotional issues will occur gradually over a period of time. If you can offer your animal treatments on a regular basis, as frequently as you are able, and be patient, you'll very likely be rewarded with some wonderful changes in your relationship and in his behavior. If you keep a journal of your animal's progress, you'll probably be surprised at the changes that are possible with Reiki. It may take a series of treatments over days,

FRAZIER: THIRTY-TWO AND GOING STRONG!

Frazier is the oldest cat at BrightHaven animal sanctuary: a senior kitty who thinks he's a teenager! His vibrant spirit and youthful disposition certainly don't match his rough exterior. He's been fighting cancer for several years now, even losing an eye from the disease, but it doesn't slow him down!

Frazier is quite the character when it comes to Reiki. He not only asks for it, he *demands* it. As soon as I arrive, I'll feel his paws scratching at my legs. As soon as we make eye contact, Frazier begins meowing. When I begin treatment, he just settles on my lap and relaxes. Sometimes he falls asleep, but many times, he just lies quietly, intently focused on the energy he's absorbing. Occasionally he'll have a healing reaction, in which he'll begin sneezing (possibly due to the tumor in his face) but soon he settles down again, taking a deep breath and burrowing into my lap.

Frazier moves around a lot during hands-on treatments, directing my hand to different parts of his body. He likes to feel treatments directly on the parts of his body that are most uncomfortable. For example, he often pushes his head into my hands (not usually a comfortable position for most cats!). No matter how long I do Reiki with Frazier (sometimes he sits with me for more than two hours), he always wants more. When I leave, he sits quietly, watching my retreating footsteps with an expression on his face that says, "Come back soon, please." —*Kathleen*

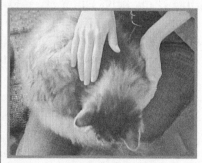

Frazier turns his body slightly so that Kathleen's hands will center over his shoulders and chest.

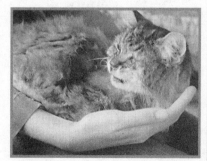

Frazier adjusts his position so that his face (where his tumor is located) is directly in Kathleen's hands.

SWENSON: THE ULTIMATE THOROUGHBRED

Swenson is a beautiful 23-year-old Thoroughbred, a racehorse in his youth. He's now my trainer Alison's school horse, and what a school horse he is! He has taught all ages of riders all kinds of skills, from flat work to jumping. He has even taught me a few things, including helping me build my confidence. Alison has had him almost 20 years, and in their youth together, they had quite a show jumping career.

Twelve years ago, Swenson became terribly ill: his equilibrium was off and he would start spinning in circles uncontrollably before lying down. His local vet was treating him symptomatically to try to get him well enough to travel to the hospital. Alison slept at the barn every night, watching over him. Her veterinarian warned that if he began violently seizuring, he would have to be euthanized. During this time, Alison's father began to give him Reiki treatments. In about a month, his balance had returned to him and he was able to travel to the hospital. The vets who examined him there couldn't believe it was the same horse that had been so sick in the weeks before the visit. He was so well in fact, they told Alison she could begin bringing him back to work.

Alison believes he was brought back by the combination of Western medicine and Reiki treatments Alison's father gave. Thus, when I moved to the barn

weeks, months or occasionally even years, depending on the severity of the issues your animal is facing.

■ Overview of the treatment

The approach As with all animals, but especially with our frailest animal friends, asking permission and letting them know they need only take the energy they want is a must.

Treating from a distance Begin at a distance and pay attention to your animal's wishes about how he wants Reiki. If you notice him settling down nearby, maybe even falling asleep as you send Reiki, this is a sign that he's accepting the energy you are offering.

Basic body positions Only use hands-on Reiki when your animal asks for it. Reiki is just as effective when given from one or two positions for the whole treatment so don't feel you have to move your hands if your animal has settled comfortably into the treatment. If you think moving your hands will disturb him or wake him up, just keep them in one place for as long as seems most comfortable for him.

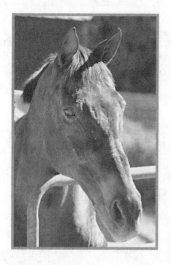

with Shawnee, Alison immediately wanted me to begin giving Swenson Reiki. So, Swenson has been my Reiki client for over two years now, receiving regular weekly treatments.

Swenson has always been very open to receiving Reiki, especially on his lower back, which gets sore now and again. He actually turns his body around, pushing his sore areas into my hands. Swenson usually falls asleep during his Reiki treatments, often lowering his head with his tongue hanging out.

I'm sure that Swenson doesn't concern himself with his age. And he's in such great shape that he looks and acts like a youngster. He truly loves to work, and as he gets older, he just gets wiser. He absolutely loves the kids who take lessons on him, and I can't imagine he'll ever give up this important job. I know that Reiki is supporting him and helping him move forward as he wishes to, full steam ahead! —*Kathleen*

Extra positions Pay attention to the areas of greatest need: these may be physical (and your animal may place certain parts of his body into your hands for treatment) or they may be mental/spiritual (and you may get intuition about what these issues are). You can trust Reiki to go to the issues of healing your animal needs most, whether or not you know exactly what these issues are. Remember, using Reiki regularly with your animal will help develop your intuition about what's going on with your animal.

Finishing the treatment Remember to thank Reiki for the healing it has brought and to thank your animal for his participation. You may want to spend a few minutes with him for affection, scratches or pats, depending on what he enjoys, at the end of the treatment to reaffirm your bond with each other.

(see Chapters 4 and 5 for further information)

▬ Hands-on treatment

Give animals the choice to come to you, rather than you approaching them for treatments. Joey, the "guardian" of the Bright-

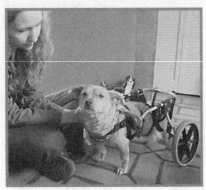

Joey shows Kathleen where he wants the healing energy.

Haven animal sanctuary, is a perfect example: If you were to follow him around, trying to force him to sit down for a Reiki treatment, he would run all over the house avoiding you. In stark contrast, if you just place yourself in a room nearby and ask his permission, waiting patiently in a place easily accessible to his

wheelchair, Joey will come right over for some hands-on Reiki.

Frazier, another BrightHaven resident, will signal his desire for a Reiki treatment by scratching at your pants leg and meowing. You can then pick him up into your lap and he immediately settles in for a long hands-on treatment.

You also need to let the animal choose how the treatment will unfold. In the picture on this page, Joey places the parts of his body he wants Kathleen to touch into her hands. He then places the front of his body near her lap and becomes extremely relaxed. Kathleen ends the treatment and thanks Joey for choosing to participate in his own healing process.

chapter 15

Reiki with Wild Animals

WILD ANIMALS ARE INCREDIBLE TEACHERS of Reiki and of the possibilities within relationships between people and animals. Their willingness to enter into a partnership for healing with humans shows the enormous potential of Reiki for animals and its benefits in promoting harmony with other species. With all animals, the more you can let go of your preconceptions about their intelligence and what they are capable of thinking and feeling, the more successful you'll be in establishing relationships with them, including relationships for the purpose of healing. Wild animals will sense when your mind is open to new possibilities with them and will be more at ease with you as they are accorded more respect.

You can use Reiki to heal the injured wild animals that cross your path, and they may begin to present themselves to you more often when they sense the healing energy you offer. If a wild animal lives somewhere around your home, you can offer him Reiki as a gift, to enhance his health and ability to function in the wild and as a way of getting to know him better. Most of the guidelines for companion ani-

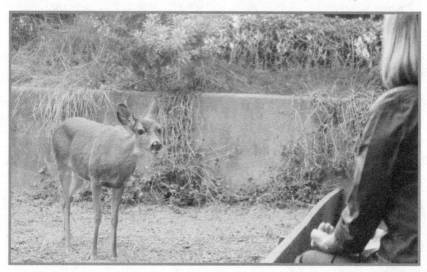

THE PHOTO SHOOT

Over the past five years I've sent Reiki to the deer and other wild animals in my neighborhood to help them deal with the many challenges of living in a suburban environment. The deer face a lot of hardships: finding food, avoiding cars and dogs, and dealing with hostility from people. They have felt the healing energy I sent, and gradually we have moved into a close relationship. They have come to trust me and to regard me as their healer. Whenever they are sick or injured, they come to my entry courtyard and wait until I come home or until I look out and see them there. Sometimes they even go from window to window, looking in to try to catch my attention if I'm home.

Over time they have brought all manner of injuries and illnesses to me for treatment. When a deer comes for help, I sit quietly in the courtyard with my hands in my lap and let the Reiki energy flow to him. Each deer decides how he wants to receive the treatment, moving around the courtyard as he sees fit and leaving when he has had enough Reiki. If I don't know why a deer is seeking Reiki, I never worry because I know Reiki will go where it's needed, whether I know what this is or not.

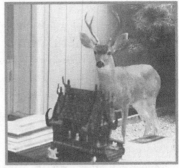

My work with the deer and other wild animals has taught me more about animals and healing than anything else I have done or read. Their understanding of Reiki and their incorporation of it into the life of the herd are, to me, the ultimate testimonials to its potential for animals. And for me, living and working with wild animals is the realization of a childhood dream of understanding, affection and mutual support with wild creatures.

Merlin looks in the window for Elizabeth.

When I scheduled the photo shoot for this chapter, I was unsure how the deer would respond to the presence of a photographer. They're accustomed to my being alone when I offer them Reiki, and I wondered if they'd be comfortable

mals apply to wild animals as well. The major exception is that truly wild animals rarely seek hands-on treatments.

As with any animal, you'll be much more likely to have a successful and rewarding interaction if you explain what you're doing and ask him to take only the amount of healing energy that he wishes to receive. It can be especially important with wild animals to make it clear that you are only offering Reiki to them, and it's up to them to decide whether

enough to show the relationship they have with me and with Reiki in the presence of a strange person and with the unfamiliar noise of a camera.

On the day before the shoot, I sent Reiki to the situation and asked the deer to come the following day at the appointed time. I told them how much I would like for them to be in the book, especially since they have been such important teachers for me, but I stressed that I wanted them to do only what was comfortable for them and would understand if participating was not comfortable. I tried to set aside any expectations and trust that in the long run what happened when the photographer came would be right for me, the deer and the book.

The next day when I came home from lunch, I was encouraged to find the grand stag, Achilles, resting on the ledge in the courtyard, two hours early for our appointment. Later, just before the photographer arrived, I went outside and found that there were now a dozen deer waiting for me. The usual way that treatments unfold was turned around that day. Normally the deer will come alone for a treatment. I had never done a group treatment with the deer, and they had never sought Reiki without a clear need of their own for it.

When the photographer arrived, the deer were calm and focused. Over the next hour and a half they took turns seeking treatment. They accommodated each other beautifully, with the majority waiting patiently off to the side and out of the way of the photos or on the ledge until each deer was finished with Reiki and it was time for the next deer to step in. The deer's desire to help me gave me enormous joy and, as we worked together and Reiki filled the courtyard, I could feel the excitement and delight rising for all of us—the deer, the photographer and me—as the shoot continued to unfold.

After we had completed the deer photos, we moved inside, expecting that we had completed all the photos of wild animals that we would get that day. However, the squirrel, Reepicheep, surprised me by waiting on the deck to offer his participation as well. Reep was uncertain about the photographer. He was too uneasy to stay for the full length of a normal treatment, but he stayed long enough to contribute some lovely photos of a treatment of a squirrel. At the end of the shoot I felt that Reep and the deer had really extended themselves to help Reiki reach other animals and to give something back to me and to Reiki for what they have received in the past. —*Elizabeth*

they wish to receive it and how much they wish to have. You'll be able to tell whether the animal accepts your offer by the feeling of energy flowing in your hands as well by the animal's body language and the relaxation they will often display.

Wild animals, such as deer, raccoons, bears and skunks, often live in close proximity with humans, trying to survive in a rapidly diminishing habitat. People may see these wild neighbors as anything from lovely additions to the scenery to annoying or even dangerous visitors that wreak havoc on their gardens and property. Using Reiki with the wild animals around your home is a wonderful way to help them to heal, to get to know them better, to deepen your understanding of their unique "survival wisdom" and undomesticated natures, and to appreciate the gifts and talents that allow them to live and flourish, generation after generation, within human civilization. In addition, using Reiki with wild animals can bring harmony to your relationship with them.

Other wild animals who will benefit from Reiki are those no longer living in the wild. These animals have found themselves in captivity, through illness or injury (such as birds or marine animals in sanctuaries and rehabilitation or rescue centers) or for other reasons, such as those who find themselves in zoos, aquariums or circuses. Many are bred into captivity, establishing long lineages of "wild" animals who haven't been free for generations. In addition to healing injuries and illnesses, Reiki can help captive wild animals to find greater

MERLIN

One day near the beginning of my experiences with deer, I noticed that one of the young stags was limping. When I got a closer look at his right hind leg,

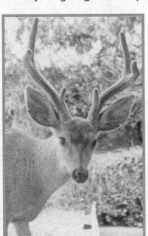

I could see a large, swollen, infected area above the hock and extending down below it. There were several long, open, festering wounds there, similar to the kind of lacerations animals sometimes get from being tangled in barbed wire. It looked as though it had been there for some time.

I sat down and offered him Reiki, which he accepted gratefully. Off and on when I saw him, and when I thought of it outside of his presence, I sent Reiki to him, and, in a couple of weeks his wound had healed. He began to come more frequently to my courtyard and a special friendship developed between us. He was the first deer to whom I gave a name, Merlin. Merlin has weathered many injuries, including one that almost ended his life. Each time he has come to me, and I'll never be able to express how much his trust has meant to me. —*Elizabeth*

BACK TO THE FOREST

One late summer day a few years ago, I was by myself in a beautiful forest on the slope of Mt. Shasta in northern California. It was an exquisite day with perfect weather, and I sat down on a rock to savor all of the beauty around me. I decided spontaneously to send Reiki to the forest around me to give something back to the forest for the joy and peace it was giving me.

I let myself drift inward into the meditative state Reiki often induces, but from time to time I opened my eyes and took in what was going on around me. The first time I opened my eyes, a butterfly that was hovering nearby came over and landed on my knee. The next time, a dragonfly hovering stayed in close proximity to me. While I was sitting on the rock and sending Reiki, I could hear a chipmunk skittering back and forth from tree to tree nearby. After a while I realized that I had not heard him for some time. When I opened my eyes, the chipmunk was about five feet away, sitting quietly with a dreamy expression on his face. Experiences like this have shown me many times how easily animals recognize the healing nature of Reiki and how strongly they're drawn to its gentle power. —*Elizabeth*

contentment and satisfaction in their lives. Using Reiki with these animals, who have lost their freedom and connection with the wild world, is a way to bring healing to their situations individually and to human relationships with animals as a whole.

Using Reiki at local sanctuaries and wildlife centers can help sick or injured animals heal more quickly and support their release back into the wild. Reiki can bring peace and comfort for the animals who must remain in captivity. Reiki can heal the memories of abuse that some animals hold, allowing them to move forward to a more joyful future.

If you volunteer your Reiki services to the animals in these settings, you can sit outside their enclosures to treat them. If you visit your local zoo or aquarium, you can sit on a bench outside the animal's cage or tank and offer Reiki to the animals from a distance. Even though you make no physical contact, the animals will show signs of appreciation such as yawning, resting or even falling asleep. Like other animals, they'll often offer gestures of gratitude for the healing you give them.

If you have Level 2 Reiki, you can heal situations that arise concerning wildlife. When sending

Reiki for this purpose, you can simply focus on the situation that concerns you. For example, if the raccoons near your house have been waking you up at night with their noise, you could focus on "keeping the peace" between you and them by asking them to make less noise near your house at night and sending Reiki for the situation to resolve so that you and the raccoons can live in harmony.

With Level 2 Reiki you can also send mental and emotional healing to wild animals, for instance, to aid an animal who has lost a much-loved companion or mate. You can send Reiki to promote harmony between your companion animals and the wild ones living nearby as well. You can also send Reiki to broader issues that speak to you, such as the loss or pollution of habitat of many species or the international trade in endangered species. You can send Reiki to open people's hearts and help them to grow in compassion and respect for the wild ones who share this planet with us.

Using Reiki with wild animals can bring you a deeper understanding of the level of intelligence and emotion that these animals possess. A relationship with wild animals through Reiki brings a new understanding of the possibilities for the future of man's relationship to his wild cousins. These possibilities include coexistence in harmony and an acknowledgement of their rights to exist in an adequate habitat and to be treated with respect and dignity. Reiki with wild animals not only heals them but heals our hearts as well by helping us remember that we're all aspects of one world and that what happens to one of us affects all of us. By observing them and listening to their needs, we learn a surprising amount about how to heal ourselves and our world.

▬ Overview of the treatment

The approach Always begin by asking the animal to take only the amount of energy that he wishes to have and allowing him to choose whether or not to have a treatment. Let him know that he's in control of the treatment.

Treating from a distance Begin by sitting at a safe distance from the animal if you feel he'll be able to tolerate your presence, or outside his presence if you feel he'll be uncomfortable with you nearby. Wild animals may not stay long for a treatment the first time it's offered. They may, however, be more receptive to subsequent offers of Reiki and may even seek out healing on their own. Always use caution with wild animals, especially if they're injured, remembering that Reiki is equally effective when offered from a distance. One of the reasons Reiki is a wonderful healing

COMMUNICATING WITH RACCOONS

When my husband and I moved into our house, we were told by the previous owners that there was a family of raccoons that lived under the shed, and that they were often out in the backyard in the early evening, running around and playing with each other. This bothered me since we have a dog, and I didn't want there to be any skirmishes with the raccoons. In addition, we had been losing sleep due to raccoon fights taking place outside our bedroom window.

One day I stood outside the shed and offered a distant treatment for the raccoons and the situation. I introduced myself to the raccoons, told them we were the new owners of the house, told them that I understood and respected that they had been here longer than we had, and told them that they were welcome to stay. I warned them that we had a dog and that they should not come out during the day. I promised that at night I would walk my dog in the front yard only. I also told them that I didn't want to hear any late-night fighting with other animals or skirmishes under our bedroom window. That night and every night for about a week, I sent the same message with a distant treatment. Interestingly, I never saw or heard anything from the raccoons, and I wondered if perhaps they had moved somewhere else.

About five months after we moved in, we had to replace the back fence after it blew down during a storm. The workmen came in and in one day removed the back fence, dug and cemented holes for the posts, and stacked up the wood for completing the repair the next day. That night, just at twilight, I was in my kitchen doing dishes and looked out the window to see a huge raccoon walking back and forth along the fence line, touching and smelling the posts, and surveying what change had taken place. I was surprised that he was still living under the shed, and I realized that my Reiki message had been received.

This spring I decided to go into the shed to reorganize some of the boxes I kept there. As I banged around at 10 a.m., I heard the loud trilling of several raccoons, obviously awakened by my noise. I mentally sent them an apology and finished my work as quietly as possible. As soon as I quieted down, they settled into silence again. I was amazed that not only did our shed house that huge raccoon, but also some babies! I thanked them for keeping to themselves as I had asked, and told them they were welcome to stay. —*Kathleen*

ASRIEL

One day early in my association with the deer, I came home from running errands and found a mature and regal stag, with an enormous rack of antlers, resting on the ledge at the far end of my entry courtyard. As I looked through my purse for my keys, I could hear loud rumblings from his belly and then a belch. As I went in and out unloading packages, the noises continued, and it seemed as though he was having quite a bout of indigestion. I had a little time so I sat down inside and offered him a short Level 2 Reiki treatment.

I got drawn into the treatment, and it turned out to be longer than I planned. When it was over, I went to the door and softly opened it to see how the stag was doing. He was asleep on the ledge; at the click of the latch, his head shot up with the most surprised expression on his face, as though he was thinking, "How did I end up asleep here on the ledge in the middle of the day?" It was his first introduction to Reiki. After this he became a regular visitor to the courtyard, and I gave him the name Asriel, after the character in the Philip Pullman books, because of his strength and his powerful presence. —*Elizabeth*

method for wild animals is that it can be done at a distance, preserving a "comfort zone" between you and the animal.

Finishing the treatment Watch the animal's body language and tune into the flow of the Reiki energy to tell when the treatment is coming to an end. The treatment is coming to an end when an animal comes out of a state of deep relaxation or sleep, moves away and becomes occupied with something else, or the energy in your hands decreases or settles at a lower level. Remember to thank Reiki for the healing it has brought and to thank the animal for his participation. Wild animals also offer their thanks, often by making sustained eye contact

or stretching in your direction after a treatment.

(see Chapters 4 and 5 for further information)

■ Treating from a distance

Most wild animals appreciate the healing energy of Reiki and prefer Reiki from a distance, as illustrated in the following story.

On the day of the photo shoot, a dozen wild deer gathered in Elizabeth's entry courtyard and on the ledge above it. She sat down quietly, put her hands in her lap, and offered Reiki to any of the deer who wished to have it (picture 1 on page 149). Elizabeth remained seated, quietly sending Reiki, while the deer decided how the treatments would go.

Calm and focused, Athena was the first to volunteer (picture 2 on page 149). Athena hopped down off the ledge and let it be known she wanted to be first by standing in front of Elizabeth and engaging Elizabeth very directly with her eyes.

As the treatment continued, Athena shifted from time to time to position different areas of her body closest to Elizabeth for Reiki. As shown in picture 3 on page 149, Athena wanted Reiki for her left side. Toward the end of the treatment, Athena relaxed and dozed.

When Athena was finished, she stretched her head out toward Elizabeth in a gesture of gratitude for the healing. Her big, soft eyes said thank you quite eloquently (see picture on page 141).

After Athena's treatment ended, several deer milled around while they decided who would go next. Diana, another doe, decided to take the next treatment. About eight other deer stood just outside the photo throughout most of the treat-

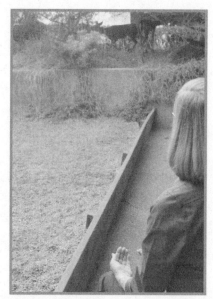

1. Elizabeth offers Reiki to the deer gathered in the entry courtyard.

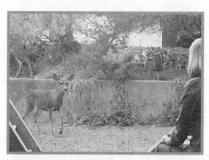

2. Athena agrees to Reiki and approaches.

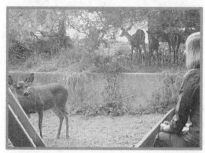

3. Athena repositions herself to show Elizabeth where she wants Reiki.

ments, watching the proceedings and thinking about whether they wanted treatments as well.

Diana wanted Reiki for her hind end for most of her treatment. She shifted several times to place her hind quarters nearer to Elizabeth. She dozed and chewed her cud, a sign of relaxation for deer. By the end of the treatment, she had turned and was dozing with her back and hind quarters toward Elizabeth, taking quite a lot of Reiki.

Diana had almost finished her treatment when the stag, Achilles, decided it was his turn and chased her off. He had been waiting patiently, but suddenly it was time for his treatment! Achilles had an old injury in his

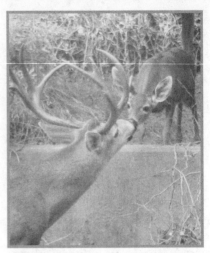

Achilles touches noses with a fawn at the end of his treatment.

front left leg and held it up. He dozed awhile and, as he woke up, he scratched his nose on his leg. Then he touched his nose very sweetly to that of the fawn who had been waiting, jumped up on the ledge and bounded off, his treatment finished.

The fawn tried to be next, but the young stag, Siddhartha, had other ideas and chased her away so he could have a treatment. Siddhartha stayed in one place and took a short treatment before we had to end the photo shoot and call it a day. Elizabeth thanked all the deer and felt tremendous gratitude to them for all they had done to demonstrate what can happen when you offer Reiki to wild animals.

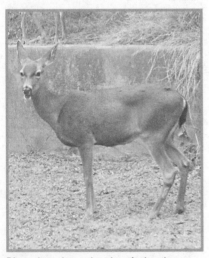

Diana chews her cud, a sign of relaxation.

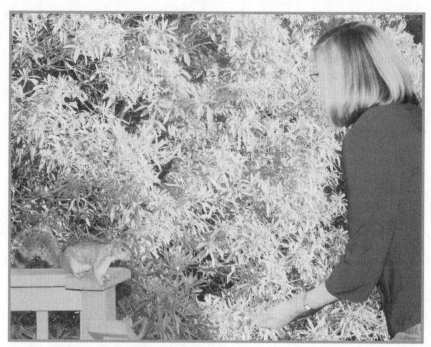
Elizabeth offers Reiki to Reepicheep the squirrel.

Soon after this, Reepicheep the squirrel approached Elizabeth for Reiki. She held out her hands and let the Reiki energy flow to Reep, who checked out the photographer to decide whether it was safe to risk a treatment. Then Reep investigated the energy coming from Elizabeth's hands. Elizabeth remained in one place, eventually sitting down to be more comfortable while offering Reiki to him. Eventually, continuing to have doubts about the photographer, Reep cut short his treatment. He held Elizabeth's gaze deeply for a moment to say thank you and goodbye before he scampered off.

▬ Hands-on treatment

Wild animals who have had regular contact with people, such as those in sanctuaries, sometimes seek out hands-on Reiki by moving close to you or placing themselves under your hands. If a wild animal moves close to you, it's generally a sign of trust, but unless he makes physical contact with you himself, he is probably not seeking hands-on Reiki.

If the animal initiates contact with you, place your hands where they seem most comfortable for him, directly on his body or several inches away. For larger animals, the shoulder is often a good place to start a hands-on treatment. The photos in Chapter 10: Reiki for Horses show a series of hand positions that work well for many large animals in maintaining health and treating an injury or illness.

chapter 16

Reiki with Dying Animals

The whole family, human and animal alike, is deeply affected when an animal member is dying. Reiki is a gentle and powerful way to support the entire family as it goes through the process of losing a beloved member. It helps to bring peace to everyone and to the overall situation surrounding the death. Reiki given at or near the time of death can bring about emotional and spiritual healing for the animal and his family, as well as acceptance and relief from pain and fear for the animal during the process.

People often feel helpless when an animal approaches his transition and wish there was more they could do to assist their beloved friend. Reiki can help you provide for many of your animal's needs at the end of his life, including physical comfort and emotional and spiritual support. Reiki can improve the quality of your animal's life—

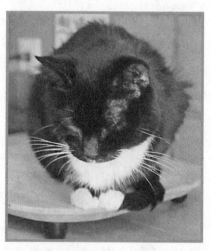

many animals show relief of symptoms and an improvement in mood and spirit. Some animals may even live longer, in comfort and joy, than anyone has expected. For others, Reiki makes passing easier, and assists the spirit in moving on after death.

The ideal approach is to begin treatments early in the process and continue them through the animal's transition. However, we have often observed that Reiki will provide what is needed most within the time that is available for it to do its work. We have seen even one treatment bring about extraordinary shifts in a situation and help an animal and his family experience his transition with peace and acceptance.

A FAMILY FINDS PEACE

I first met Karson the cat about two weeks before his transition. He and his family were in a state of extreme exhaustion and worry. Karson had had cancer for nearly a year and had been unable to get comfortable and sleep for quite a while; his doting family woke when he did and spent their nights trying to help him and worrying about him. He had enjoyed a wonderful life with them and there was enormous love between them.

Karson's family loved him deeply and was having a great deal of difficulty accepting that he was dying and that he was, in fact, quite close to making his transition. He was holding on as best he could but was very worried about them and whether they would be all right without him, and he was not sure he could hang on until they were able to understand that he was ready to leave this world. They were taking him to the vet frequently for more treatments and diagnostic tests and trying new medications, and Karson was beyond the point at which this was doing him any good; he wished they'd stop and accept that his time was very limited. He was concerned about what would happen to them when he passed on because they seemed unable to accept the inevitability of his death.

During his first treatment it took Karson quite a while to decide whether Reiki was going to be a good thing. He moved around the house for about 20 minutes but eventually he settled into one place near my hands and absorbed a great deal of energy. Afterward he and his family slept peacefully for about a week and they reported that he seemed much more comfortable.

When he became uncomfortable again, they had me back for another treatment. At this point Karson was not sleeping and was having difficulty moving around, preferring to lie in one place all the time. As soon as I arrived he came

Although the end of life inevitably brings sadness, many beautiful things can happen during this period. People who have used Reiki with their animals at this time often say they grew closer as the transition grew near. The inevitable grief at separation can be tempered by the sense of fulfillment accompanying a deeper bond at the end.

Healing does not always mean cure

Using Reiki with dying animals can be very challenging. As healers, we want so much for the animal to get well, and we can feel discouraged if the animal is not able to do so. Reiki provides each being with the healing that's most needed within the frame-

over and climbed onto my chest, where he remained for an hour and a half, absorbing an enormous amount of Reiki. His family was amazed because he never climbed onto anyone outside the family before. Along with healing, I sent Reiki to his situation with the hope that his family would be able to accept his condition and the nearness and inevitability of his death. That afternoon and evening he was able to move around the house in his accustomed way: he was able to go into the back yard and sit on the front porch again at sunset, as had once been his daily habit. He was more comfortable, alert and interactive with his loved ones.

When I came back a couple of days later, they had accepted his condition and stopped all veterinary interventions except those to make him more comfortable at home. They wanted to learn Reiki so they could assist him as much as possible in his last days and to help them with their grief when he passed on. Since my next class was a week away and I didn't feel Karson would live that long, we started Reiki lessons at their home that day. Karson was present for the classes that day and the next. As we finished up the lessons, he was nauseated and beginning to be in discomfort, but he insisted on being present with his special person during the last initiation. I left after the initiation. Within an hour, his condition deteriorated rapidly, and they took him to the emergency clinic where they decided it would be best to assist him with euthanasia. They said that he passed on peacefully with a big smile on his face at the end.

Soon afterward his family wrote to say that they weren't grieving as severely as they had thought they would. They felt they had done well at the end and that Karson was in a good place now and wouldn't want them to grieve excessively. They had devised some practices, such as lighting candles daily on his grave and making a photo album of their time together, that gave them comfort and closure. —*Elizabeth*

work of that being's destiny. For this reason, healing doesn't always mean cure. We always remind ourselves that Reiki always works for the highest good of the animal, even when the result isn't what we hoped for. In retrospect, we can usually see how Reiki brought healing to a situation and often why this was the healing that was needed most.

Sometimes when people learn Reiki to help their own terminally ill animal or treat a dying animal soon after learning Reiki, they can become discouraged and challenged in their belief in Reiki when they are unable to prevent the transition. An animal apparently on the verge of death will sometimes recover with Reiki; in these cases, it seems that, despite how dire the situation may have become, it's not truly the animal's time to transition, and Reiki can restore him to health.

If it's an animal's time to leave this world, Reiki won't prevent the transition, although it can greatly ease the transition between life and death. In this case, it frequently acts by enhancing the quality of life, by shifting the situation so that all concerned can accept the transition and let go with greater ease, and by enabling the transition to be easier and accompanied by less suffering. Reiki will provide dying animals and their families with the support that's needed, easing pain and fear and helping the animal to make the transition with peace and acceptance.

If we allow ourselves to focus on physical recovery as the only evidence that healing has taken place, we may find ourselves feeling helpless and discouraged if the animal passes away. It helps to remember that death is a natural part of life and that offering Reiki to an animal during his transition is a wonderful, loving gift that can bring healing on emotional and spiritual levels. We know that we can trust Reiki.

THE MOUSE

One day as I was coming home, I interrupted my cat Emma as she was finishing off a mouse in our courtyard. When I put Emma inside and returned to the mouse, he lay completely motionless with a large drop of blood coming from a puncture wound on his back. It looked as though Emma had finished the job before I got to her, but something inside me said to try Reiki all the same.

I sat down on the doorstep and sent Reiki to the mouse, who lay about a foot away. I was pulled deeply into the treatment and did not realize how much time was passing. When I looked at my watch, 30 minutes had passed and the mouse still lay exactly as Emma had left him. I was tempted to stop, but again something said, "Go on a little longer." After a few more minutes the mouse twitched and soon stood up and looked around, holding my gaze for a few seconds. Then he ran across the courtyard and disappeared into the ivy.

Later that day I looked in the ivy, hoping I wouldn't see a little mouse body, and I didn't. The next day, as I was sending Reiki to the deer, a little mouse, identical to the one from the day before, took a couple of steps away from the ivy and looked at me for a minute. I like to think that he was the near-casualty of the day before, checking back with me to say "thank you." —*Elizabeth*

A MOMENT OF PEACE

Sometimes an animal's circumstances cannot be changed, but Reiki can bring healing to any situation. One dog I worked on had suffered such abuse and terror at human hands that she was completely vicious and untouchable. She was on the euthanasia list, so I decided to offer her Reiki for her situation. I strove to keep my emotional center serene and mentally let her know that I was offering her healing, if she chose to accept it. I asked for Highest Good, hoping for a miracle to save her life, if that was possible.

Although she refused to lie down or even sit, she eventually leaned her body against the wall of the kennel, hung her head low to the ground, and closed her eyes. I felt peace and harmony surrounding both of us; my head felt far away, as if we were all alone in another world. This quiet place lasted for about ten minutes. During my subsequent visit to the shelter, I learned that she had been euthanized. This was difficult for me to hear, but I remembered how peaceful she had been during the treatment. Reflecting on the peace and harmony surrounding us then, I felt she received healing on a spiritual level so that she was ready to make her transition. —*Kathleen*

In a loving and compassionate way, Reiki always brings the healing the animal needs. We may not always be aware of all of the issues the animal is facing, but the healing will always occur.

It is a tremendous gift to be able to bring relief and comfort to your animal, to be peaceful enough to allow him to go through the process in his own way, and perhaps even to be with him, sending healing energy, as he makes his transition. Through it all, Reiki will surround you with healing, comfort and a gentle peace. The greatest gift of using Reiki to help your animal pass on is the deepened understanding of the dying process you'll receive and the inner peace you'll achieve because of this.

How to begin

Dying animals are sometimes more sensitive to energy and other stimuli than they had been earlier in their lives. Even animals who formerly delighted in hands-on Reiki will sometimes begin to prefer Reiki at a distance as they near the end of their lives. Each animal is an individual, and some will prefer to be closer to you, even preferring hands-on treatments when in the past they preferred treatments at a distance.

HELPING A HORSE LET GO

Sometimes dying animals will seek out Reiki on their own. One such horse was an old Arab gelding with whom I had little contact, except the occasional hello, since he lived in the same stable as my own horse. From others in the barn, I knew he was suffering pain and very, very old. One evening, I was mixing warm water into my horse's grain at a sink adjacent to the arena where the old horse was standing. Because of his lack of mobility, he was allowed to roam free there. Out of the corner of my eye, I saw the old boy slowly walking towards me, head lowered, eyes fixed on me. As soon as our eyes met, I absolutely understood that he wanted Reiki. As soon as I mentally agreed to give him Reiki, he lay down and stretched his head down onto the ground. I squatted down about 20 feet away and offered Reiki. He closed his eyes and gave a deep sigh.

My head felt thick, sleepy and very light all at the same time. It often feels that way when I work with dying animals, as if they're already separated from their physical bodies. Gladly, I felt no pain or anxiety from him at all. He showed no signs of even being aware or concerned about the horses or people around. It was as if he was just so tired, so exhausted, and so ready to let go.

So it's best to start by offering Reiki to your animal from a short distance and watching for signs of his preference. If he can't get up and come to you for hands-on Reiki, he may stretch his neck toward you or do something else to indicate that he would like you to draw closer. Tuning in to your own intuition is valuable, since you know your animal better than anyone and can probably read his signals quite well to discern what his preference is about Reiki.

As soon as you intend for the Reiki to flow to your animal, the treatment will begin. You may feel an intense flow of Reiki or only a mild flow, and you may be drawn deeply inward or find yourself talking and communing with your animal throughout the treatment. If your animal indicates that he would like hands-on Reiki, you can follow his lead regarding placement of your hands. At times putting your hands on areas affected by his illness or injury may be uncomfortable for him, and he'll prefer them on an unaffected area; at other times, your hands may be soothing and provide relief from pain or other symptoms. Each treatment may not be exactly like the last one, and you may need to

I sent Reiki to his situation for the highest good and decided to stop the treatment as a small, worried crowd began to gather. The horse's people arrived with the vet and cleared the barn, asking everyone to leave. As I drove away, I felt helpless. I prayed that Reiki would facilitate what the horse needed. Later that night, I got a call from a friend. The old horse had been euthanized. Apparently it was a difficult decision for the horse's people. It could have gone either way, but the decision to help him pass was made. They were all together when he passed.

I was so relieved! I sent Reiki to his spirit that night, holding the intention that his passing was peaceful and easy. The next day when I walked past the place where he lay the night before, I felt the old horse's presence very strongly. I acknowledged his spirit, thanked him for his openness to Reiki, and told him it was okay to move on when he was ready. As I look back on this experience, I feel truly grateful to have been a part of the process, even if in a small way. Although I know it was difficult for his people to help him pass on, I had clearly felt from the horse that it was his time. Before this experience, I wasn't sure if euthanasia could ever be a peaceful way to go. Now I feel sure that sometimes, it's exactly what an animal needs. Reiki never ceases to amaze me how it can smooth the way, whatever that way may be. —*Kathleen*

experiment carefully to see what is best for your animal in the current treatment.

Each treatment can be a special time between you. The treatment will be coming to an end when you feel the flow of Reiki begin to taper off or when your animal moves away or shows signs of turning his attention to something else. Sometimes the flow of Reiki will continue indefinitely, and you'll have to stop the treatment for your own reasons.

In offering Reiki to your beloved animal in his last days, you'll often experience profound and life-changing lessons. You can give Reiki to your animal as he approaches his transition, as he's dying and even afterward. Reiki can improve the quality of your animal's life while he's living, make his passing easier, and assist his spirit in moving on after death. With Reiki given at the end of life, many animals show relief of symptoms and an improvement in mood and spirit. Some animals may even live longer, in comfort and joy, than anyone has expected.

Giving yourself and other family members (both animal and human) Reiki during this

REMEMBERING CRYSTAL

I met Crystal in a Reiki class I taught at BrightHaven animal sanctuary. She jumped into my lap, curled herself into a ball, and settled in for a long treatment. While usually I circulate around the area, checking on students' progress, I found myself instead giving a Reiki treatment to Crystal. When the students returned to discuss their results, Crystal stayed. In fact, she refused to move from my lap for over two hours. When I had to leave for the day, she grudgingly allowed herself to be gently placed on the couch, but looked questioningly at me as if to say, "And when will you be back?"

So I did return to give her some treatments, especially when I heard that she was approaching her transition. One particular day I found her napping on the bathroom counter, and noticed how in just a few weeks' time she looked much more frail. In fact, I was afraid to disturb her so I just settled quietly in a nearby chair and asked permission to begin the treatment. She woke up and lifted her head. When she recognized me, she immediately got up and tried to jump into my lap for hands-on Reiki. I couldn't believe the motivation she suddenly showed! I quickly got up so I could gently place her in my lap (despite her obvious enthusiasm, I wasn't sure she would physically be able to do it on her own). Again, she settled into a deep sleep for over an hour. When I finally had to leave, I had to pry her again from my lap. I told her I'd send her regular distant treatments to help her.

On June 15, 2005, Crystal passed away peacefully in Gail's arms. Gail, her person, was also able to offer her regular Reiki treatments as Crystal's life came to a close. She shared with me later that Reiki was the only thing that gave Crystal physical comfort in her last days. She said she could see in her eyes the peace and comfort Reiki brought. —*Kathleen*

time is also very beneficial, as it will help you heal fear and worry about the transition process. Being able to feel more at peace with your animal's passing will allow you to be truly present with him in his last days and moments and will help you to make decisions with more clarity. It will also help your animal's passing be easier for him. Often animals take our worry and fear upon themselves to help us. They can be at peace with their own transition process but become concerned about our anxiety. When they see that we are at peace and "OK," they are often able to turn inward and focus on their own dying process. Sending Reiki to yourself, or having a friend send Reiki to you, after your animal's transition can be a tremendous help in coping with the inevitable grief that accompanies separation from a beloved friend.

■ Overview of the treatment

Starting from a distance   It's best to start by offering Reiki to your animal from a short distance and allow him to approach you if he wants hands-on Reiki. Dying animals are sometimes more sensitive to energy and other stimuli than they had been earlier in their lives, so you should take extra care in watching for your animal's preference. For example, if he can't get up and come to you for hands-on Reiki, he may stretch his neck toward you or do something else to indicate that he'd like you to come closer.

Keep in mind: Begin by letting your animal know that he can choose whether or not to receive a treatment and how much Reiki he wants to take. Watch your animal's body language and tune into the flow of energy in your hands and your intuition to determine how he wants to have the treatment.

Possible hand positions   If your animal indicates that he'd like hands-on Reiki, follow his lead regarding placement of your hands. Keep in mind that, at times, putting your hands on areas affected by his illness or injury may be uncomfortable for him; at other times, your hands may be soothing or provide relief from pain or other symptoms. Each treatment may not unfold exactly like the last one, so proceed carefully to see what's best for your animal at that time.

Finishing the treatment   The treatment will be ending when you feel the flow of Reiki lessen and your animal begins to show signs that he's finished with the treatment. Remember to thank Reiki for the healing and to give

HOSPICE, SANCTUARY AND SHELTER SUPPORT

Reiki is a tremendous addition to any hospice program for animals. It's also a valuable skill for the staff at shelters, sanctuaries and rescue organizations, or any setting where aging or terminally ill animals may be present or where euthanasia is practiced. Even one treatment can make a great difference in the experience an animal has in transition. In shelters where euthanasia is practiced, giving Reiki to animals who are scheduled for euthanasia is a priceless gift. Being able to offer this form of compassionate assistance to animals scheduled for euthanasia helps shelter staff members as well and can reduce the burn-out they sometimes experience in their jobs.

your animal love and gratitude for his part in the treatment.

(see Chapters 4 and 5 for further information)

▬ The greatest gift

Animals can be among our most beloved and closest confidantes, and losing one of them is as painful as losing a human family member. Animals often sense their people's anxiety about losing them and hold on longer than they would like in order to spare their people the pain of loss and to give them time to adjust to their passing. Although you may wish for a miraculous physical cure when you are facing the death of a loved one, sometimes there are deeper levels of healing needed and more profound lessons to be learned. As one dog with cancer and his family beautifully illustrated, although Reiki may not always cure disease on the physical level, wonderful healing shifts on the spiritual and emotional levels can take place. With Reiki, death can be a peaceful process, and sometimes the greatest gift of healing you can give an animal is just to let them go from this life, with love and acceptance.

Melissa brought Elizabeth and Kathleen her 110-pound Malamute, Misha, because he had advanced bone cancer in his shoulder. She was trying to decide whether to amputate the leg as the doctors had recommended

MICK: HEALING BODY AND SPIRIT

When I first met Mick, a resident of BrightHaven animal sanctuary, he was so depressed, it was heartbreaking. He suffered from chronic irritable bowel disorder, and had recently been having a series of ups and downs physically. Some of the volunteers at BrightHaven wondered if he was nearing his transition. That particular day, he was in a lot of pain. His eyes were glazed over and he showed no interest in my (or anyone else's, for that matter,) presence. Before I began the Reiki, he wouldn't even lie down, and was standing around, looking uncomfortable. I sat in a chair about ten feet from where he was standing so as not to invade his space, and asked his permission to begin the treatment. Almost immediately after I began the treatment, he lay down, closed his eyes, and fell into a deep sleep: his feet even ran in a kitty dream at one point!

After about 30 minutes, he woke up and opened his eyes: His eyes were bright and focused, and he looked straight at me and meowed quietly. He even

and wanted to try Reiki to help her with making the decision and to see if it could help Misha. She was having difficulty facing the seriousness of his condition and was hoping for a physical miracle. Along with Misha, she brought her other dog, Buddy, a brown toy poodle who was both blind and deaf. Elizabeth and Kathleen ended up offering the treatment to Misha out on the front lawn, as this was the only place he seemed comfortable.

Almost as soon as the treatment began, Elizabeth felt enormous sadness coming from Misha, which brought tears to her eyes. At the same time, Kathleen began feeling extremely nauseated and asked Melissa if Misha had been feeling sick to his stomach. She replied that his stomach had seemed fine, but a few moments later Buddy (who had been wandering around a few feet away) began vomiting. At this point Elizabeth and Kathleen realized that Buddy, despite being blind and deaf, knew exactly what was going on in his family, and was extremely anxious about it. They asked Melissa how the family had been doing with Misha's illness, and she confirmed that the whole family had been highly stressed and saddened by the illness and pain Misha was going through. Elizabeth and Kathleen decided to offer a distant treatment on the situation for the entire family: Melissa, the two dogs and two cats, who were at home.

allowed me to pet him a bit as I thanked him for being open to the treatment (and he could be quite temperamental, so this was a great honor!).

After this initial treatment, Mick received several more Reiki treatments, both in person and distantly, from both me and one of the BrightHaven volunteers. He soaked up the Reiki like a sponge every time. He began to gain weight and improve physically, and his spirits raised dramatically. Gail (the founder of BrightHaven) joked with me that Reiki had backfired: Mick was so much his old self that he was once again stealing food from other cats and making himself an utter nuisance!

The last time I saw Mick, I was making a short visit to BrightHaven. When I came in the front door, I saw Mick across the room and called his name. He saw me and bounded across the floor, happily pushing his face into my hands. Quickly he turned and bounded off. I was surprised and delighted by his exuberance. A few days later, Mick's spirit left his tiny body as he was cradled by Gail and surrounded by his BrightHaven family. —*Kathleen*

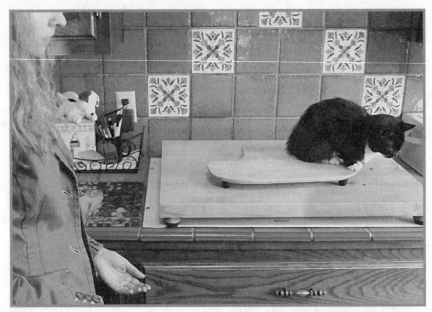

Mick has irritable bowel disease, and hands-on Reiki feels too intense for him. With regular treatments from a distance, however, he has chosen to accept Reiki, gained weight and found comfort and relief. Here, Kathleen has placed herself nearby, but not in Mick's physical space. He becomes relaxed and rests, with his eyes closed, during the treatment.

As soon as the treatment for the family situation began, the energy shifted and became lighter. Buddy stopped vomiting and settled down to rest. Melissa began to throw carrot sticks to Misha, who joyfully caught and ate each one. Both were smiling. It was a beautiful and peaceful picture, their worry and pain forgotten in the enjoyment of the moment.

Discussing the treatment with Kathleen later, Elizabeth shared the intuitive communication she received from Misha. He let her know that he felt absolutely responsible for this family. He felt such a tremendous sense of duty and loyalty for them that he was holding on for them, despite the pain. He was waiting for his family to come to terms with his condition so he could transition peacefully, with their support and acceptance. We hoped that the emotional shift we had witnessed would continue on after the treatment.

A few months later, Elizabeth and Kathleen heard from Melissa again. She related that things had really seemed to turn around after the treatment. The morning after the treatment she had felt clear that she should go ahead with the amputation. Wonderfully, afterward, Misha had been mobile and relatively pain-free until very recently. A few days before her call, he had lain down and been unable to get up, and his bodily functions were closing down. She said that she had finally been able to come to terms with the fact that his time on this earth was ending, and felt that it'd be kindest to help him with his transition with euthanasia. However, she wasn't sure whether it was the right time, and hoped a Reiki treatment would help clarify things.

Elizabeth and Kathleen met Misha again in a park near the Golden Gate Bridge on a beautiful day: sunny, windy, and warm with a slight chill in the air. When they arrived, he lay on a white blanket in the grass under a tree. He seemed to recognize Elizabeth and Kathleen, although they reintroduced themselves to him. They began to offer Reiki to both Misha and the family situation, and asked Reiki for gentle and compassionate healing for the highest good. Misha immediately

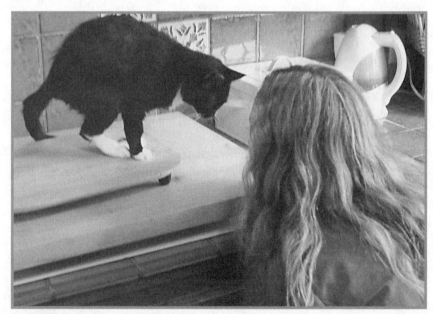

Cats often tell you when they're done with the treatment. Here, he gets up and stretches. Kathleen spends a few moments to say thank you and tell him how special he is before she leaves.

laid his head on the grass and sighed, as if welcoming the healing energy. Elizabeth and Kathleen both went very deeply into the treatment, feeling very light and at peace, as if the physical world were very far away.

About 45 minutes into the treatment, Kathleen began to feel tightness in her chest, which turned to heaviness, then pain, then anxiety, causing her legs to shake and teeth to chatter. She immediately realized that this was not her own anxiety, but information received from Misha. Kathleen mentally thanked Misha for sharing this with her, and told him she was listening to him if he had anything to share.

Her intuition told her he was asking the question, "Is it okay to let go?" She shared this question with Melissa. Melissa, speaking clearly and honestly from her heart, began to tell her beloved dog that it was okay for him to go, and that although she would miss him greatly, she'd be all right. Simultaneously, Kathleen began to have deep breaths, one upon the other, as the flow of Reiki increased. They weren't sudden and sharp breaths, but rather long, slow and deep. A few moments later, as her breathing became

normal again, Kathleen's feelings of anxiety from Misha were replaced by a deep sense of peace.

Misha lifted his head and made deep, soulful eye contact with us, as if to say "Thank you," and with that it seemed that the treatment was over. Elizabeth and Kathleen thanked Misha for sharing so much, and Reiki for healing and guiding with such love and lightness.

In this second treatment with Misha, Elizabeth and Kathleen felt another definite shift in the energy of the situation: a feeling of acceptance, peace and clarity for Melissa and Misha. They felt that Reiki had helped in the process of letting go. As they left, Melissa and Misha lay together face to face in the grass, really listening to and understanding each other. It was a truly touching and beautiful moment; Elizabeth and Kathleen felt honored to be a part of their healing process, and very at peace with the outcome of the treatment.

During the treatment, Reiki had surrounded Elizabeth and Kathleen with such a feeling of peace and comfort that they felt certain that the highest good in the healing process had been served. Melissa later said that Misha passed away very peacefully the next day. His family had been able to grieve without being overwhelmed, and they were recovering and going on with their lives, just as Misha would've wanted. Although the family had initially sought a miracle on the physical level, Reiki brought them a miracle of a different kind: a miracle of healing through peace, acceptance and the ability to let go.

Expanding Your Reiki Journey

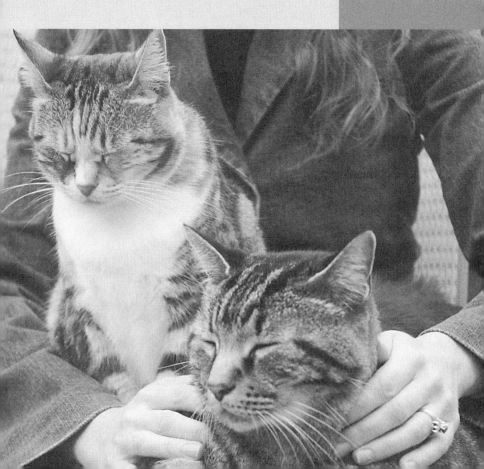

Part Four

chapter 17

Offering Reiki to Animals beyond Your Own Animal Family

WITH ANY LEVEL OF REIKI you choose to learn, there are different scopes of practice you may be drawn to. Some people treat only themselves and their own animal companions. Some people may be drawn to healing only friends, family and the animals within this circle. Others wish to offer healing beyond their intimate circle to strangers, animals they do not know, and situations beyond their immediate experience. There are also different levels of frequency of Reiki practice. Some people practice only occasionally; others practice often or even daily, and some establish a professional practice of Reiki. Regardless of the scope and frequency of practice chosen, Reiki will enhance your life and the lives of those around you.

For those who want to expand their practice of Reiki beyond their own animal family, there are a few additional matters to consider as you begin to offer Reiki to animals and people you may not know well.

▄▄ Communicating with the animal's companion before the treatment

Before you begin a treatment with an animal, it's a good idea to talk with his human companion about what Reiki is and how you'll be giving the treatment. People's ideas about Reiki can vary widely, and it can be helpful to have a short discussion of what you'll be doing and why so that the person knows what to expect.

Try to be careful about what you discuss about the animal in his presence. Animals understand much more than most people realize, picking up on body language, emotions and often even pictures and images in our minds. Having an emotional discussion about the animal's health in his presence can cause him undue stress and fear. When you discuss his health situation with his person in his presence, try to do so with discretion and compassion so as not to frighten the animal.

Once the treatment begins, it's better to cease conversation until the treatment ends. If the animal's person wishes to be present during the treatment, he can sit quietly, read, meditate or otherwise remain quiet. If possible, he should also avoid actively engaging his animal because this will impede relaxation.

■ Meeting an animal for the first time

When meeting an animal for the first time, strive to appear and behave in a way that inspires trust and doesn't overly excite the animal since you'll want him to be able to relax deeply into the treatment you're about to give. Sometimes people bring food or a treat to an animal as an offering of friendship, but it's best to refrain from bringing food when your purpose is to give Reiki, as it can be an incredible distraction. You want the animal to think of you as the "Reiki person," not the "treat person."

You want the animal's first impression of you to be of someone who is interested and attuned to him, who will listen to him and take his needs and concerns into account. A quiet, calm manner

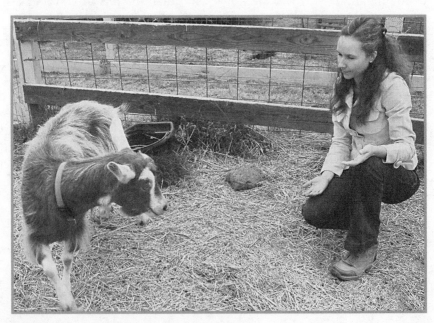

and voice and still, gentle hands help to convey this impression.

Some animals seem more relaxed if they can see your eyes, so you may want to remove your sunglasses before you go in to give a treatment. Also, hats can sometimes be frightening to animals, especially dogs. In general, animals are more sensitive to smells than humans are, so try to avoid perfume and other strongly scented products when preparing to give a treatment. However, if you need to use hats or sunglasses or have other physical issues, try to be as present, centered, calm and sensitive as possible. This is the state that will inspire the most trust, thus setting the stage for a successful treatment.

▰ Communicating with the animal

It's important to take a positive approach in communicating directly with the animal. Allow animals who are in pain, frightened or upset to express their feelings while offering a positive form of encouragement or reassurance. For instance, telling them "You're safe here; I'm here to help you" is more reassuring than "Don't be scared, no one will hurt you." In the first sen-
tence the animal is likely to pick up the images and feeling tone of the key words "safe" and "help"; in the latter, he may pick up images and feelings associated with "scared" and "hurt."

In communicating with animals, it's important never to promise something you can't deliver or tell an animal something that isn't true. Honesty breeds trust and respect is vital to animal communication and healing. Animals sense when our emotions aren't congruent with the communication we're sending them; the more simple, positive and authentic our communications are, the more successful we will be in communicating with animals and in strengthening our bond with them.

▰ Working with aggressive animals

Always be careful to conduct treatments under safe conditions. Maintain a safe distance when giving Reiki to an animal that may be aggressive or potentially dangerous and make sure there is a barrier between you and the animal, if necessary. Try not to stare at the animal or react strongly to any lunging or snarling he may exhibit during the treatment. Strive to maintain a calm and centered attitude. If you sense that the animal will feel invaded by direct communication with you, keep a respectful mental distance from the animal and ask Reiki to work for the highest good. As always, ask Reiki to give the animal only what he's willing to take.

Eventually even the most aggressive animals will usually accept a Reiki treatment for at least a brief period. However, if the animal continues to resist the treatment, you should stop and try again another day or you can try offering healing outside his presence with Level 2 distant Reiki (see Chapters 18 and 19). A distant treatment will almost always be acceptable to the animal, but if, after a short period of trying, it isn't, then the animal's wishes should be respected and you should stop trying to send Reiki directly to the animal. A Level 2 distant treatment could be sent to his situation instead.

▬ Communicating with the animal's companion after the treatment

At times, the insights you receive during a treatment can be helpful to share with the animal's person so that he can better understand the animal's condition and how he can be of help to his animal. However, it takes some experience to effectively communicate the information you receive to the animal's person, and it's always best to use as much discretion and compassion as possible in this regard.

It's important to remember that animals' human companions are always doing the best that they can at any given time. If you can show them something about their animal or their relationship with the animal in a caring and compassionate manner and without judging or criticizing, you may be able to help them. It's never helpful to convey information in a critical manner or make an animal's companion feel bad about his actions. Since animals are usually closely attuned to their person's emotional state, causing distress to the person will also be distressing to the animal and will, in all likelihood, cause him to withdraw from the healing relationship with you.

Sometimes it's better to keep some or all of the insights you receive to yourself if you feel that the person won't be able to understand them or if you feel you lack the skill to communicate them effectively to the animal's person. An alternative approach, which is very effective and can do no harm, is to send Level 2 distant Reiki healing to the relationship between the animal and person or to the animal's situation with the person (see Chapters 18 and 19). This approach can bring about positive shifts without causing distress to any party. The healing can be sent to the relationship or situation in general, without further specification, and the innate wisdom of Reiki will heal the situation in the way that's needed most.

The communications the animal sends you will help him even if you don't share them with his person. You're a supportive presence and a witness as the animal revisits and releases emotions that have been pent up and unresolved within the safe situation of a Reiki treatment. Releasing these old emotional issues frees the animal to move on into his present and future, no longer burdened by the past, lighter in heart and more open to the relationships and events of the present moment.

chapter 18

Level 2 Reiki

WITH LEVEL 2 REIKI, you'll become acquainted with the full range of Reiki healing available to animals. Level 2 Reiki expands the circumstances under which treatments can be given to animals and the depth of the healing that can be obtained with Reiki treatments. The ability to heal more deeply at the mental, emotional and spiritual levels brings new dimensions of healing to animals and enables you to deepen your own healing journey as well.

Several characteristics differentiate Level 2 Reiki from Level 1 Reiki:

- The Reiki energy that flows through you is stronger, reaches more deeply and intensifies self-healing and the healing of others.

- Healing can be sent across distances, great or small, to the intended recipient; with Level 2 Reiki, this can include situations as well as individuals and groups.

- Deeper mental, emotional and spiritual healing can be achieved.

Two new types of treatments become possible at Level 2: the distant treatment and the mental healing treatment. This chapter and the following chapter will focus on these two new types of treatments.

■■ Three symbols

At Level 2, the Reiki student learns three ancient symbols that can be used to increase the healing power of the energy, to focus treatments on mental and emotional issues, and to heal from a distance. These symbols function like keys that unlock the expanded capabilities of Level 2 Reiki. While we describe the symbols and their uses in a general way in the following sections, the Level 2 symbols and the specific details of how to use them are sacred and powerful; in our view they should be kept private and used with respect and discretion. The specifics of how to use the symbols is learned in a Level 2 class. Our focus is the ways in which Level 2 Reiki can be used with animals

THE POWER SYMBOL

The power symbol is used to increase the power and flow of the Reiki energy and, therefore, the strength of the treatment given. It's used in healing serious problems or in any situation where you want to use the maximum healing available to you. It can also be used to increase the speed with which the energy flows so that more healing can be delivered in a shorter period of time. When the power symbol is used, you'll often feel the flow of energy through you increase.

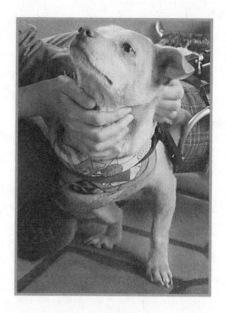

In addition to the basic uses taught in a Level 2 class, the power symbol can be used alone in many creative ways. For example, you can use the power symbol at the beginning of a treatment to increase the power of the energy sent throughout the whole treatment. Or the symbol can be used directly over a part of the body that needs extra healing. You can draw the symbol on your palm and then place your palm directly on the part of the body that needs healing. Or it can be drawn on a towel, cloth or other object that can be placed under, over or near a sick person

or animal to provide continuous, gentle support and healing.

The power symbol can be used alone as a protective barrier, placed in front of or spiraled around an animal or person in need of protection. It can also be drawn and sent mentally to any situation or being that's in need of help or healing. It can be used to clear the energy of a room or of new objects brought into a space. It can be drawn over medicines, herbs, flower essences or essential oils to increase their effectiveness. It can be drawn over water or food to enhance their supportive and nutritive qualities. As your experience grows, you'll often find new and exciting ways to use this symbol.

THE ELEPHANT WHO DIDN'T FORGET

One of my distant clients was an elephant who had, after more than 35 years in a zoo, finally found a wonderful sanctuary in which to live. She had occasionally shown aggression to handlers in her past but had been very docile 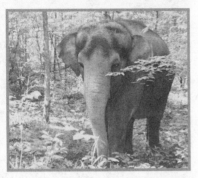 since coming to the sanctuary, where she was given respect and freedom of choice, and was allowed to roam freely over hundreds of wooded acres. After visiting the sanctuary, I found myself thinking about her one day, especially about her life as a young elephant. I decided to offer her distant Reiki to heal her past.

Immediately as I began the treatment, I felt an extremely strong flow of energy. In fact, my dog came across the room and lay at my feet, which he sometimes does to absorb Reiki during a really strong treatment. After about ten minutes, I suddenly got the very strong picture of concrete floors with pools of water on them. Simultaneously, my eyes began to water, the tears running down my face uncontrollably. It felt as though the flow of energy would never end, and it was a very long treatment.

When I contacted the elephant's caregiver, she was very interested in the picture I had received. She told me that the elephant had been kept most of her life in a terrible indoor room that had wet concrete floors. I was very amazed, and realized that I had received a memory from the elephant during the Reiki treatment. I felt sure that Reiki was facilitating the healing process of this elephant's past. —*Kathleen*

After drawing the power symbol, you'll often feel increased physical sensations in your hands or body as the flow of energy through you increases. When the power symbol is used in treating your animal, he'll sometimes feel the increase in energy and may look at you with increased interest or even with surprise. Your animal may twitch or yawn as the energy flows more strongly to the area that needs healing and may relax more fully into the treatment.

THE MENTAL HEALING SYMBOL

The mental healing symbol is used to focus healing on mental, emotional and spiritual issues. Many animals have mental or emotional difficulties, such as aggression, anxiety, depression or withdrawal, as a result of previous trauma, abuse, loss or grief. Many behavioral issues also have roots in mental and emotional issues. Physical issues can have mental, emotional or spiritual causes as well. These difficulties often improve rapidly when a mental healing is given. The mental healing symbol reaches deeply into the animal or person receiving a treatment, connecting directly with the mind, emotions and spirit of the recipient and bringing deep healing. For this reason it must be used with great care and respect with each animal.

As with all treatments, in giving a mental healing to your animal, always leave it up to him to determine whether he chooses to have a mental healing and how much healing he wants to receive. You can do this by asking your animal at the beginning of the treatment to take only the degree of mental, emotional and spiritual healing he's willing to accept. If you feel he's not willing to receive a mental healing directly, you can send a treatment to his general situation instead. Because animals can't always tell you what's bothering them or what lies at the root of their challenges, the mental healing symbol can be the most potent and useful tool of the animal Reiki

practitioner. However, its use should always be guided by the strictest ethical considerations, including those concerning the animal's freedom of choice in receiving a Reiki treatment.

Using the mental healing symbol can bring mental clarity and healing to animals by bringing unresolved matters to the surface when this is in the best interest of the animal. This symbol can access the higher spiritual self of the animal to change patterns and bring about healing on a deep level. It can accelerate mental, emotional and spiritual healing by allowing the animal to acknowledge, honor and release blockages that have prevented healing. He can then move on in

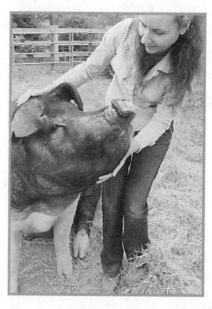

his journey with a lighter heart and be more open to the positive possibilities available to him in the present and future.

THE DISTANT SYMBOL

Because it's pure energy, Reiki isn't subject to the limitations of time or space. We are all made up of and connected by energy and our energy fields interact with each other at all times. With Reiki, the healing energy of the universe flows through the practitioner and along the energetic pathways and connections all around us to the intended recipient. With Level 1 Reiki, this heal-ing can travel in close proximity; with Level 2 Reiki, healing can travel across a room, to the other side of the world, or even into the past or future. Level 2 distant treatments are just as effective as treatments given in person.

Ever since Einstein's Theory of Relativity was embraced by the scientific community, scientists have accepted that space and time are relative, not absolute, concepts, and this concept is basic to the field of quantum physics. Although science cannot yet explain phenomena like Reiki in concrete terms, the conceptual

MERLIN SHARES HIS HEART

I often go into a treatment thinking one thing needs healing, and come out of it with a very different sense of the situation. One such experience was with a woman named Kay who sought Reiki for her horse for self-inflicted scratches and cuts. Merlin was 17 years old and a high-level dressage horse. At the time, Kay hadn't been his person for very long and couldn't figure out why he kept hurting himself.

Although outwardly it appeared that the treatment should be focused on the scratches and cuts on his legs, as soon as I started, I began to get feelings of intense anxiety and sadness from Merlin. I had a strong feeling that he was worried that if he disappointed his person, she would sell him. I had the intu-ition that this had happened before. I thanked him for sharing these feelings with me, and let him know that I understood what he was feeling. Immedi-ately, he moved his body into my hands, leaning his chest into my palms. He seemed relieved that he could share this with me and that I was listening.

Shortly thereafter, he turned around and went to the back of his stall as far away from me as possible. This is a common reaction after an animal shares an intense emotion. He needed his space after the close connection he made with me. I continued to offer Reiki from a distance of several feet away, not invad-

framework necessary to do so in the future has been expanding for many years. It's just a matter of time until scientists will be able to explain how energy can travel across time and space, and thus give us a window into the workings of Level 2 Reiki.

However, because it's so esoteric, Level 2 Reiki is usually easier to learn when the student has become experienced and comfortable with Level 1 Reiki. For many people, learning Level 1 Reiki introduces many new ideas and possibilities that they've never considered before; these ideas are often enough to occupy their thoughts initially without adding the concepts of Level 2 as well.

When first introduced to Level 2 Reiki, some people have a hard time believing that they can send healing effectively across distance and time. They feel as though this idea is going against everything they've been taught by society, including beliefs about the nature of time and space, about how beings and objects affect each other, and about the effect of intention on beings and situations outside one's immediate physical vicinity.

ing his space. By the end of the treatment, he had returned to my hands again, the anxiety and sadness had subsided, and he felt much calmer and more peaceful. After I finished the treatment, he turned to face me and lightly touched his muzzle to each of my palms, first the right hand and then the left. Then he put his nose to my chest and sighed. It was one of the most exquisite thank-yous I've ever received.

I gave Merlin a series of four treatments for his injuries, emotional healing and his situation. I also spoke with Kay about his deep anxiety and fear that he would disappoint her if he couldn't work for her and that he might lose her. Soon afterwards, she realized that due to hard training in his past before she had him, he had such severe arthritis that he needed to retire.

Making this decision was very difficult for her. However, as soon as she told him not only that he could retire but also that she'd always look after him and take care of him no matter what, there was an incredible lift in the horse's spirit and calm in his eye. After many years, he had finally found his special person, who would value him for his essence as a being rather than his ability to perform. It was wonderful to see the healing of the bond between this horse and his human! Although Merlin has recently made his transition, Kay gave him a great gift: during the last part of his life, he knew he was cherished for who he was, not merely for what he could do. —*Kathleen*

COMFORT TO A CAT

Toodles was an orange tabby cat much loved by her mom Janet, a coworker of mine. She worked with ferals and we often shared animal stories with each other. I knew her kitty was getting on in years and suffering from congestive heart failure, but he seemed to be holding on. One day Janet came in to work really upset because he had taken a turn for the worse. His digestion had completely stopped and he was so agitated that she was unable to hydrate him as the vet had shown her. I went home immediately after work, focused on a picture of him, and sent him a Reiki treatment. The next day, Janet was grateful. Toodles was so calm the evening before that she had no trouble hydrating him, and he started going to the bathroom again. She was also happily surprised that Reiki could work so well distantly. Although Toodles has since made his transition, Reiki helped improve his quality of life by lessening his physical discomfort. —*Kathleen*

By suspending their doubts and beginning to use Level 2 Reiki, however, they learn through their own experiences that this kind of healing is possible. Kathleen's experience is a good example.

When Kathleen first learned Level 2 Reiki, she had fortunately experienced enough positive healing situations in her own life from Level 1 Reiki that she was able to continue practicing distant healing, even though she wondered at first if the treatments were effective. As she sent distant Reiki, she would get feelings of pain and buzzing in her hands or head that she would usually ignore. After a while, she realized that these sensations were clues about what needed healing in whatever she was sending Reiki to.

Kathleen started sending treatments to friends and family over a far distance, calling them afterwards or the next day to check in. She questioned them about what she had felt when giving the treatment, like, "Is your left knee bothering you?" or "Are you feeling anxious about something?" Incredibly, the answers absolutely confirmed her own experiences when giving the treatment. Still, each time Kathleen got confirmation, she doubted that it could happen again and thought that perhaps it was a coincidence. With more and more distant treatments given, however, her confidence in Reiki's power beyond "hands on" grew by leaps and bounds.

Soon Kathleen began to give treatments to friends of friends, people she didn't know anything about. Still Reiki showed her the way, revealing whatever information could help her in understanding the healing process. She began to think of unconventional ways to use distant Reiki for healing in her own life. Soon, Kathleen was sending Reiki to her childhood difficulties, her negative life-patterns, and even her future. Each time she sent Reiki, she felt a shift in energy, an unfolding of the true process of healing.

When Kathleen worked with animals, however, she still relied upon a hands-on approach. When animals would be restless or unapproachable, she got frustrated or believed that the animal didn't want Reiki. Somewhere along the way, a light bulb went on and she decided to try distant Reiki with animals. She found that it was easier to do a combination of hands-on and distant Reiki because then the animal had the freedom to move around. She no longer had that nagging thought that she needed to restrict the movement of the animal. The animals were thankful, even if she never entered their cage or paddock. She also often sent Reiki to the animal's past and future during these treatments.

Kathleen began to do distant Reiki in her yard: to the tree, the roses, the ivy, whatever came to mind. When a honeybee or yellow jacket would fly by, she

BAILEY REBOUNDS TO HEALTH

Bailey is a seven-year-old cat who lives with his family in Detroit. He suffered from recurrent asthma and bronchitis, and his person Jill wanted to try Reiki to see if it could help him with his illness. I sent a series of treatments to Bailey over several months, and his condition began to improve almost immediately.

Bailey had experienced a great deal of hardship and grief before he came to Jill. And, as Jill and I talked about the treatments over a period of a month or so, Jill remembered that she had had a difficult time in her early life as well and carried a number of emotional scars from the past. She decided to re-examine the issues from her past and sought professional help in understanding and releasing them. I sent Reiki to Jill and Bailey together to help them release the effects of old trauma. As Jill examined her past and gained new understanding of it, Bailey's health continued to improve. The last time I heard from them, Bailey had been well for many months, and Jill felt everyone in their family was benefiting from their improved health. —*Elizabeth*

would send Reiki and blessings to it. Often they would linger nearby, buzzing in circles around her.

Eventually Kathleen realized that all creatures and beings felt Reiki and loved it. Even now, every day, she finds new ways to use distant Reiki to bring healing to herself, other beings, and the world around her. She's still always amazed at the results distant Reiki can bring to beings and situations.

Distant Reiki generally feels less intense to animals and can be more comfortable for those who are especially sensitive to energy. It's often ideal for animals who are wild, very small, fearful of strangers, old, fragile or close to death. They can often relax and absorb Reiki more easily and comfortably when treatments are given distantly. It's also ideal in situations where it's inadvisable or impossible to be close to or have physical contact with an animal, such as when working with unpredictable or aggressive animals, with wild animals, or with animals that live at great distances from the practitioner.

Distant treatments have many uses and open up a whole new world of possibilities with Reiki. They can be sent to individual beings, to groups or to situations. They can be sent to a being directly beside you or on the other side of the world. They can be sent to the past and future. They can be sent to situations in which you are participating, situ-

SANCTUARY FOUND

One day as I was leaving the shelter, one of the employees approached me about her concern over a Rottweiler. His aggression problems made him unadoptable. She told me that he had been scheduled to be euthanized two days before, but due to an employee's illness, it had been put on hold. She had been trying to find a sanctuary with no luck. She said she couldn't even look him in the eyes because he seemed to know his time was up and looked terribly forlorn.

That week I sent Reiki to his situation for his highest good, that if possible a miracle could save him, or that his passing would be quick and gentle should he be put down. The following week on my visit to the shelter, I learned that at the last minute, the day after this treatment, a sanctuary had been found that could take him in a month, and that in the meantime they had found a boarding facility that agreed to keep him. —*Kathleen*

GRETA AND HER FAMILY GET BETTER TOGETHER

Greta is a beautiful little gray-and-caramel-colored cat, quite petite and full of kittenish exuberance despite her eight years. One of her people, Claire, had heard me speak at a workshop about the advantages of working with an animal's whole family when it's possible. Working with the whole family benefits everyone; it helps the animal to achieve greater improvement by helping his people to heal, thereby shifting important elements of his emotional environment and allowing for greater change.

Claire requested a series of distant treatments for Greta's chronic digestive symptoms and wanted me to send Reiki for herself and her partner as well. Greta loved her treatments immediately and, after five or six treatments, Claire reported that Greta's symptoms had improved and that she and her partner had also made some shifts, individually and together, that were benefiting all three of them. They continue to seek out treatments on a regular basis to maintain and increase their gains. —*Elizabeth*

ations you witness, or even situations outside of your direct experience. Distant Reiki can be sent simultaneously to an animal and to his person or to the situation surrounding the animal. The distant healing symbol can be used to open the doors of time and space, allowing you to direct healing to an animal's past and future, to send healing from a distance, and to direct healing to all aspects of an animal's situation.

When using Level 2 Reiki, because of the power, depth and range of the healing involved, it's useful for the practitioner to remind herself of her position as merely the channel of Reiki energy by asking for divine order or highest good for the healing

process. In many situations, it's impossible for the practitioner to know what is best for the animal, but Reiki will always heal for the best. Remember, as in any Reiki treatment, always ask permission from your animal client before you begin.

▄▄ Level 2 benefits to animals

Level 2 Reiki offers the same benefits to animals as Reiki given hands-on or from a short distance, but it greatly expands the range of animals that can be treated, the circumstances in which they can be treated, and the depth of healing that can be obtained. For example, a Level 2 Reiki treatment can provide the

HORACE IS FINALLY HEARD

A year ago I was contacted by Cathy, whose cat Horace had an inoperable tumor in his throat and was approaching his transition. She wanted me to come to her house and give him a series of Reiki treatments to help him with his transition. As we ended the call, she added, with considerable embarrassment, that she had a major "pack rat problem" and was being monitored by the city because of her tendency to accumulate belongings and her inability to let go of them. She hoped that I would still be willing to come to her home to help her cat after hearing about her "problem." I assured her I would.

When I arrived at her home I found that it was immaculately clean but stacked almost from floor to ceiling with belongings. Everything was packed neatly in plastic bins and bags and labeled, but the sheer volume of belongings was indeed unusual. Horace was resting on a towel on the couch, and as soon as I sat down he climbed on to my lap and went to sleep with my hands on him.

Cathy and I talked quietly off and on through the treatment, and she shared some of the unhappiness she had experienced in the last ten years. Over the course of four treatments as we sat enveloped by Reiki, I learned that she had experienced many losses in her early life and in the previous decade. She had "let go" of so many important emotional attachments through tragedy that she was unable to "let go" of anything else in her life unless she was forced to do so by the city. She feared she wouldn't be able to hold onto the important memories associated with her belongings if she let them go.

same benefits as Level 1 Reiki but often at deeper levels: accelerated healing from illness, injury, surgery and emotional challenges, including behavioral issues; pain relief; health maintenance and prevention of illness; and an easier and more peaceful transition at the end of life. Distant treatments can be used to heal a traumatic event in an animal's past and to heal family situations, past and present, that involve an animal, including helping human companions during the process of an animal's transition. Send-ing Reiki to situations in the future that are expected to be difficult, such as impending surgery or a move to a new environment, helps them to resolve more quickly, easily and successfully.

Animals who live closely with human companions are very much in tune with the emotional states of their people. In their efforts to protect and take care of them, animals often take on their worries, anxieties and sometimes even their physical problems. With Level 2 Reiki,

Horace had been by her side through the last decade, sometimes as her only source of emotional support, and she was having a hard time facing the prospect of a future without him. He, too, was tortured by the necessity of leaving her, an event he was delaying by sheer force of will but knew he could not avoid much longer. He wanted me to let her know how important it was for her to let go of "old things" so that new and good things could come into her life. It was very hard for him to leave without giving her this message. In each treatment, I sent Reiki to Cathy and Horace for emotional healing.

During our last Reiki treatment I relayed Horace's message to Cathy. She heard it and thanked me, but I could tell she wasn't fully taking it in. Horace felt the same way and asked me to write the message down and send it to her. He wanted her to have it to refer to in the future after he was gone and could no longer look after her. At the same time I had the idea that photographing her belongings might give her a way to remember them and help with the process of letting go. I wasn't sure whether this idea came from Horace or from me.

I felt awkward about Horace's request but did as he asked because of the force with which the message was delivered and his urgency. Horace passed away while the letter was on its way to Cathy. For a long time I heard nothing from her. Nearly a year later she contacted me to let me know she had finally taken Horace's message to heart and had begun photographing some of her belongings and then letting them go. She had organized the photos in albums so that she could look at them when she wanted to remember. She felt she was making progress in letting go of the past as her beloved Horace had so wanted her to do. —*Elizabeth*

you can communicate to the animal that taking on these issues isn't really helpful and only causes harm to himself. You can send healing to this tendency and suggest other ways that he can contribute to his person's health and growth without damaging his own health. Elizabeth's clients, Tracy and Glen, highlight this point.

Tracy and her husband Glen were distraught because their five cats, who previously had co-existed quite harmoniously, were in a state of all-out war for six months. Although they had previously been very social and affectionate, they had withdrawn from the human members of the family and were attacking each other and spraying in the house. Tracy was especially concerned about one cat, Gabe, who had developed a stress-related intestinal disorder. Tracy and her husband were both in demanding jobs and were getting ready to sell their long-time residence. They were fatigued and under a lot of stress as well.

Elizabeth started with a series of four Reiki treatments. For the first treatment she went to Tracy and Glen's home and treated all of the cats together. During this treatment each cat showed Elizabeth how he was expressing the stress in the household. One cat hid under the bed, where he had spent much of the last six months. Another stalked him and attacked the youngest, who was still a kitten. The kitten was in constant motion, antagonizing everyone. The oldest cat attempted to impose order, swatting at the kitten and guarding the cat under the bed, but could not be everywhere at once. Gabe watched all this with sad eyes from the periphery. After the first visit Elizabeth gave the cats three more treatments on consecutive days, sending Reiki to the overall situation as well.

About a week later Tracy called to tell Elizabeth that har-

A VISIT FROM CASSY

Distant Reiki is a great way to heal your animal's past as well as your own. Sometimes this can happen during the same treatment, as I learned from a treatment I gave to my cat Cassy, who passed away several years ago. The reason for the treatment came about in an unusual way. Elizabeth had called to tell me of a mother cat she was working with who didn't trust humans after her kittens were aborted. I started thinking about the cat that I had as a child. She was fixed while pregnant, and it had never occurred to me that she may have missed her babies.

I decided to offer Reiki to Cassy and her kittens. I wondered if perhaps they had reunited in the spirit world. I hoped that Reiki would heal the pain from that situation in the past, and also that Reiki would heal my own guilt as her person who thoughtlessly allowed the situation to happen. As I began the treatment, I wondered if Cassy had ever forgiven me. Almost immediately after starting, my hands began to pulse strongly. After ten minutes or so, I began to remember the specifics of Cassy's markings: for example, how her chin was half black and half white. It had been years since I'd even looked at a picture of her, and yet it was all completely clear in my mind's eye.

My hands continued to pulse. Then, suddenly, I felt a weight on my chest and felt the unmistakable and familiar vibration of a purr resonate through my chest. I remembered that she had always liked to lay on my chest. I felt her spirit there, palpably, just like the old days. I knew instantly that she was thanking me for the Reiki, and had forgiven me. As soon as I made this realization, the purring was gone. I was left with the feeling that Reiki had reached her, and that she continues to watch over me in my healing work. —*Kathleen*

PUDDLES GETS ADOPTED

I decided to send Reiki to the adoption situation of a darling brown Dachshund, Puddles, so named because of a neurological disorder that caused her to have no control over her bladder. She seemed oblivious to her problem, running happily around the shelter's yard, grabbing and shaking toys, her weak back legs tripping all over themselves. She had such a sweet temperament, but as I left the shelter that day I sadly wondered who would adopt a dog with such a messy problem. Nevertheless, I focused on the highest good and hoped that a home would be found for her. Sure enough, Puddles was adopted that very week. —*Kathleen*

mony had been restored to the household. The cats were getting along well, once again showing their full personalities, playing and interacting with their people. She asked Elizabeth to continue to send treatments for several weeks to support the family's continued healing. Two weeks later Gabe's symptoms had disappeared, and his veterinarian was taking him off his steroids and other medications. Tracy said that seeing him play like a kitten again brought tears to her eyes. Tracy and Glen decided that the cats had been responding in part to the high level of stress that Tracy and Glen had been feeling and were bringing their attention to it by steadily increasing the level of warfare and chaos among themselves until Tracy and Glen did something about it. Glen and Tracy were taking steps to reduce their own tension and stress in the hope this would help keep the peace at home for everyone.

With Level 2 Reiki, you can help animals live closely with their people while protecting their own health so that the animals can be there at their best for their people. By letting the animal know that you're sending Reiki to heal his person and/or his situation, you can bring comfort to the animal and allow him to let go of the issues that he has been taking on. When Level 2 Reiki is sent to the animal and his person together, it can help the animal both directly and through its benefits to his human companion.

■ Deepening the bond with your animal

Using Level 2 Reiki with an animal deepens the bond between you two and increases your intuition about each other's emotional states. Your animal will often learn to seek you out for Reiki and this can become a special intimate time for the two of you. You can begin to communicate more effectively with your animal and better understand his needs. Reiki is a wonderful healing tool you can use in many different ways throughout an animal's life.

chapter 19

General Guidelines for Using Level 2 Reiki with Animals

LEVEL 2 REIKI INVOLVES the use of the symbols discussed in the previous chapter. The understanding of the use and power of these symbols grows with practice, so it's a good idea for you to give the different types of Level 2 treatments as often as possible. Over time, you'll become familiar with all of the new and exciting aspects of Reiki healing that Level 2 makes possible.

The following guidelines will provide a foundation for using Level 2 Reiki with animals. We encourage you to use them as a starting point and, as your experience increases, to allow your intuition, Reiki's innate wisdom, and the animals themselves to guide you to your own unique Reiki practice.

▬ Getting ready

The guidelines for giving treatments that we discussed in Chapters 3 and 4 also apply to Level 2 treatments. Before giving a treatment, try to be aware of your own state and take care of your own basic needs so that you can focus fully on the treatment. Center yourself and give yourself a little Reiki to help with this, if it's necessary. Whether you're in the animal's presence or not, try to find a quiet place where you'll be undisturbed, and assume a comfortable position so that you'll be able to focus on the treatment for its natural length.

Because the flow of energy is stronger at Level 2, giving a distant treatment or a mental healing often causes the practitioner to go more deeply into a meditative state. It's a good idea to set aside plenty of time for the treatment, if possible. A distant treatment will take an average of 30 minutes (or anywhere from about 20 minutes to 45 minutes). A mental healing will take an average of about 10 minutes (or anywhere from 5 minutes to 20 minutes) and can be given separately on its own or added to a full treatment given in person or distantly.

SUNSHINE FINDS A SANCTUARY

A beautiful draft-cross horse named Sunshine inspired me to try using Reiki in very creative ways. She was facing euthanasia because of her age and the financial difficulties her person had taking care of her due to her severely lame legs. I spent an afternoon giving Sunshine a Reiki treatment, which she absorbed happily, and knew as I drove home that I had to find a way to save her.

When I got home, I got on the Internet and sent a distant Reiki treatment to help me find a place for Sunshine, where she could live out her days in comfort. The chances were slim because it had to cost little or no money to place her, it had to be relatively close because of her lameness issues, and because I had heard that most sanctuaries were full. I typed in "horse sanctuaries" and went to the first site I found. Dean's Horsetown, USA was in Southern California, which was a bit of a drive for such an old girl, but I emailed them. With the email, I sent a Reiki treatment that the best for Sunshine would happen.

Amazingly, they responded that one stall had just opened up. They described their facilities and the daily care they gave their horses and I knew it was the right place for Sunshine. I described Sunshine in my next email and explained her circumstances, wondering how much it would cost to get her there. I once again sent Reiki that the financial circumstances would work out for the best. I couldn't believe it when I read the reply. Not only would they take Sunshine for free despite her physical challenges, but they would pay for her transport and even had a safe, trustworthy transportation service in mind.

The final piece of the puzzle was to convince Sunshine's person. Once again, I sent a Reiki treatment to the best of Sunshine's situation. I met her person the next day and he immediately agreed to sign her over to the sanctuary. A few days later, protected by yet another Reiki treatment for a safe transport, Sunshine made the long trip down to Southern California. Not only did she travel well, but also the first thing she did when she reached her new home was to roll over and over in the dirt. According to people who knew her well, she hadn't done that in years due to her leg problems. I sent her regular distant Reiki treatments, and she lived the last year of her life there in happiness and peace, with lots of love, carrots and attention. —*Kathleen*

Sending a treatment to a situation can be done as part of a treatment given in person or as part of a distant treatment, and doesn't usually result in a significant change in the length of the treatment.

▬ Starting the treatment

Whether you're giving the treatment from far away or in the presence of your animal, begin by mentally connecting with him. Let him know you'll be offering him Reiki to help him heal. Ask your animal to take only the amount of energy that he wants and needs and reassure him that Reiki won't be stressful or invasive.

If you're giving a treatment in person, ask him where he hurts, or what his difficulties are. If he knows, he may show you, for instance, by raising the leg that hurts, touching the problem area with his nose, or sending some form of intuitive information. Give him as much freedom of movement as possible during the treatment.

If you're giving a distant treatment outside your animal's presence, try to give the treatment at a time when the animal will be resting or when he isn't engaged in an activity that requires most of his focus and attention. This is the optimal approach because animals can rest and absorb the treatment more fully under these circumstances. If you're unable to send a treatment at the optimal time because of time zone differences, for instance, or a heavy appointment schedule, you can rest assured that your animal will still receive an adequate treatment and Reiki will go where it needs to go and heal that which is most in need of healing.

■ Signs of acceptance

In the beginning, for many people, it's easier to recognize signs of acceptance of a treatment

---

A PERFECT PAIR

On one of my visits to the shelter, I was drawn to working with Beau, an 11-year-old Corgi mix with an extremely sweet temperament and a severe limp. He had such severe problems with his back leg that he needed an expensive surgery. I sat in the kennel and held him in my lap for an hour-long Reiki treatment. Once he relaxed, he stopped shaking and fell asleep. As I held him, I offered a distant treatment for Beau's adoption situation. I focused on highest good and hoped for a wonderful family to adopt him, despite his age and leg problems. As I left the shelter, I wondered about his chances. The next week, I noticed Beau wasn't there. I nervously asked an employee where he was, hoping he hadn't been euthanized. The employee happily told me that over the weekend, an elderly man with a cane and a bad leg had come in, taken one look at Beau, and immediately adopted him. What a pair! —*Kathleen*

through an animal's body language and facial expressions. As you gain experience with Reiki and become able to discern the sensations of energy flowing through you during a treatment, you can "read" the animal's response to the treatment from the flow of energy.

With Level 2, when you're giving a distant treatment outside of the presence of the animal, you can tell whether the animal is accepting the treatment, as well as which areas are drawing the most Reiki, from the sensations of the flow of energy through you. The energy will ebb and flow, your hands will heat up, buzz, throb or pulse, and you'll feel other sensations just as you do when giving a treatment in the animal's presence. If an animal is taking a very strong flow of energy during the treatment, often you'll feel far away, deep in a meditative state.

Just as with treatments in person, during a distant treatment an animal will often get very relaxed and drowsy or fall asleep. If treatments are repeated at the same time for several days in a row, the animal's person will often report that the animal went to a favorite resting place just before the treatment was scheduled, waited and then fell asleep or dosed at the time the treatment was given. After the treat-

DISTANT REIKI GIVES CHESTER MORE TIME AND COMFORT

Jennifer heard about Reiki for animals and contacted me for a series of treatments for her cat Chester, who had an inoperable cancer in his mouth. Although she hoped for a miracle, she wanted to do all she could to make his last days comfortable if it wasn't possible for him to recover. Chester was normally shy of strangers. He would hide when new people came to visit and let his brother Douglas greet them and have all the attention. For several weeks before his treatment, he had spent most of his time hiding under the bed.

When I arrived at the house for the first treatment, Chester walked right up to me and settled down at my feet as though he had been waiting for me. Jennifer was surprised by his unusual behavior, and also by Douglas'. This time Douglas stayed in the background, not even trying to greet me, and let Chester have a long treatment uninterrupted. Douglas finally came over to say hello just before Chester had completed his treatment.

Chester remained quiet and still for the whole treatment, occasionally commenting on it with chirps and meows but mostly dozing. Afterward Jennifer

ment the animal will often show an increase in vitality, emotional health, and interaction with loved ones.

When giving a treatment out of the presence of the animal, especially a mental healing, you may receive intuitive information about an animal's emotional state or other information that will help guide the process of healing, just as you do in his presence. When a particularly strong emotion or impression is received during a treatment, it's often because the treatment has begun to facilitate the release of that emotion so that healing can take place. These emotions and impressions can be startling the first few times they happen, and it helps to remember that the information you receive isn't your own but related to the animal you're treating. You can always trust Reiki and rest assured that the information you receive is helping the healing process (see Chapter 6).

In using Reiki with your animal, your primary responsibility is to assist his healing process. The best way for you to form a relationship with your animal that will support this healing process is to respect him by giving him as much choice as possible in receiving Reiki. If you sense from the feeling, or lack of feeling, in your hands and body and the

reported that he seemed happier, at times even playful and frisky. He had returned to many of his old habits, such as meeting Jennifer at the door and resting in the open on the living room carpet. Since Jennifer lived 45 minutes away, I gave Chester a combination of distant treatments and treatments in person. Jennifer said that when it was time for his distant treatments, Chester would gather himself into a "loaf shape" with ears alert and eyes closed and remain that way for the duration of the treatment. She said that after the treatment he would stretch and chirp as if to say thanks and that he was always very affectionate with her after Reiki.

Jennifer's veterinarian was surprised by how long Chester lived with his illness. I came to see him and give him a treatment for the last time the day before his death. Although he was very weak, he crawled over and draped himself over my legs as I sat on the floor and sent him Reiki. Jennifer and I felt it was his way of saying thank you for the healing he had received. He passed away peacefully at home the next day. Jennifer was grateful to Reiki for improving the quality of Chester's life at the end and allowing him to enjoy more time with her and Douglas. —*Elizabeth*

intuitive information you receive that your animal doesn't want a treatment, stop the treatment and try again another time. Bosley, a wise white cat who lived in New York, demonstrated that even at a distance an animal can say no to a treatment and should always be given a choice.

Bosley had a cancerous tumor on her lower jaw and her health was failing. Her person Mark asked Elizabeth to send a treatment to help Bosley be as comfortable as possible in the time they had left together. When Elizabeth sat down and sent Bosley Reiki for the first time, she forgot to tell Bosley what she was doing and ask Bosley to take only the amount of energy she wanted to have. Elizabeth always began treatments this way, but on this day she skipped ahead and sent Reiki to Bosley without this important step.

It was as though Elizabeth had come up against a brick wall—absolutely nothing happened. No energy flowed, no sense of connection developed, nothing. Elizabeth quickly realized what the problem was and apologized to Bosley. Elizabeth started over, this time with respect for Bosley's autonomy, and the Reiki flowed smoothly.

▬ Hand positions

Hand positions for Level 2 distant and mental healing treat-

A REIKI NAP

Three sanctuary dogs taught me that when hands-on Reiki is too intense, distant Reiki works wonders. My mom-in-law and I volunteered at an animal sanctuary, working with dogs. The dogs were kept in large octagons, each housing 16 to 24 dogs. With hundreds of dogs, you can imagine the noise! I ended up treating three coyote-mix dogs: Birdsong, Windfeather and Running Deer. The oldest one had severe arthritis in his back legs. I tried to give him hands-on Reiki, but after a few minutes his teeth began chattering and he retreated to the outdoor area to escape Reiki. The other two dogs were very open to hands-on Reiki, but I kept worrying about the old one, shaking pitifully in the outdoor area. So I decided to try healing from a distance, intending to heal all three dogs at the same time. About five minutes later, my mom-in-law said, "Hey, is it naptime? They're all asleep!" And sure enough, I looked around and noticed that every dog in the entire octagon was fast asleep. The silence was deafening. Amazingly, Reiki gave to each dog just what he needed, in a manner he could receive comfortably, even extending beyond my intended treatment area. —*Kathleen*

STERLING THE CAT

My sister's cat Sterling is a beautiful black Persian. He lives far away, so I send him regular distant treatments. My sister initially asked me to send him treatments for his polycystic kidney disease. The vet informed her of this condition during a routine checkup and told her there was no treatment or cure for the disease. When I began sending treatments, his blood work showed that he was in the beginning stages of the disease. His blood numbers were abnormal but he showed no outward symptoms.

I began with a series of four consecutive treatments. I set up the times with my sister, offering the treatments four nights in a row at the same time each night. Beginning on the second night, my sister reported that Sterling looked forward to the treatment. Although he usually sat with her to watch television in the evenings, about the time I would send the treatment, he would go upstairs and lie down in his bed. The first night it happened, she was curious about where he was going so early, so she went up to his room and found him lying on his back, all four feet in the air, out like a light. She was quite amazed at his ability to sense when Reiki was offered to him from such a distance. In fact, she was so impressed with his response to treatments that she decided to learn Reiki, and now gives him regular treatments herself. —*Kathleen*

ments for animals vary according to what seems most useful and practical in each situation. If you have a photo of the animal, you can put your hands around or near the photo while you're sending the treatment, with the intention that the energy will flow to the animal in the photo. Alternatively, a pillow, stuffed animal, doll or other figure can be used as a surrogate to represent the animal who is receiving the treatment. Using such figures can aid in your concentration, focus and ability to interpret healing information you may receive during the treatment.

A stuffed animal large enough to allow you to place your hands in a full series of positions similar to those for treating animals hands-on is useful for treatments in which you want to receive information about the various areas of the animal's body. A smaller stuffed animal, which can be enclosed within your hands, is useful for treatments in which you want to surround the whole animal with healing energy throughout the treatment. With a surrogate of any size, you can place your hands over the parts of the animal's body that you know are in particular need of healing and send Reiki.

Using a surrogate and moving through all of the suggested positions for animal hands-on treatment will give you the same detailed information about the animal's need for healing that's available from a treatment given in person. As you move your hands through the positions, you will feel the ebb and flow of energy in each area, just as you do in a hands-on treatment. This will give you a lot of information about the animal's state of health and need for healing in the various areas of his body.

You can also use your own leg or legs as a surrogate during a treatment. This approach is useful when you want more detailed information but a surrogate isn't available. In this case, you can sit down and mentally designate one of your knees as the animal's head, the front of your thigh as the front of the body, and the back of your thigh as the back of the body. You can then move

A LONG JOURNEY HOME

Melvin and Monica (the beginning of whose story is told on page 110) were overjoyed to be able to live together in one cage at the shelter. They interacted constantly and joyfully and slept snuggled together at night. Seeing how happy they were together, I sent Reiki to their situation for the right home to come to them. Several days after, a family with four young children came into the shelter looking to adopt an animal. They settled on Melvin and Monica.

They were nice people, juggling an enormous load of responsibility, including two full-time jobs and the four children. Although they were very well-intentioned, the shelter had recently had to remove a puppy from their home because they were too busy and overwhelmed to give it all the training and care it needed. Because the people were so nice and the kids seemed to be able to adjust their behavior with Melvin and Monica when they were given guidance, the shelter allowed them to adopt the two guinea pigs.

One of the animal control officers was concerned about the placement, however, and after a couple of weeks decided to stop by the family's home and see how the guinea pigs were adjusting to their new situation. She found that the novelty of the guinea pigs seemed to have worn off for the kids, and they had been relegated to a small outdoor cage which they shared with a large rabbit. The cage was cleaned infrequently and basic pellets were provided but none of the fresh foods rabbits and guinea pigs need to balance their diets. The conditions weren't poor enough under city regulations to warrant remov-

your hands through a series of positions on the front and back of the thighs, intending for the energy to flow to the corresponding area of the animal's body.

Another alternative in giving distant treatments is to write the name or description of the animal or situation being treated on a piece of paper; the paper can then be placed between your hands or inside a box on which your hands are placed during the treatment. It's also possible to send a distant or mental healing treatment without using your hands at all, but simply with mental intention. You can visualize moving through the positions of a treatment and will often get a wealth of information this way as well. Finally, you can simply sit and send Reiki without using a surrogate or visualizing any positions and Reiki will go where it's needed.

■ Ending the treatment

When giving distant and mental healing treatments, you can tune

ing Melvin and Monica. She was glad that they had each other and noted that they stayed close together and seemed to find support in each other.

When I heard about their situation, I was very puzzled because in my experience Reiki had never failed to provide a beneficial shift in a situation. I continued to send Reiki to them from time to time and tried to trust that Reiki would bring a positive resolution when the time was right. The officer visited the family two more times in the ensuing four months and each time found the situation unchanged. After her third visit, however, the mother decided that they didn't really have the time and energy to care for so many animals and brought Melvin and Monica back to the shelter.

A couple of days before Melvin and Monica returned to the shelter, a young woman named Yumiko lost her beloved guinea pig at the end of his long, happy life. Yumiko worked for a local animal rescue organization and also ran a small guinea pig rescue organization in her home. When she stopped by the shelter and met Melvin and Monica, she was moved by their story and decided to take them home to live permanently with her as her own animal companions. Yumiko was a very gentle person, and she and her husband had no children. They doted on Melvin and Monica and the other animals in their care. In her most recent email Yumiko said that Melvin and Monica still valued each others' company above all others but had settled in well at her home and enjoyed the company of the guinea pigs who passed through on their way to good homes, through Yumiko's efforts. Although it was a long and somewhat zigzag journey for them, I felt that Melvin and Monica had finally found the perfect home with Reiki's gentle assistance. —*Elizabeth*

IMPROVING BOO'S QUALITY OF LIFE

One of my clients was a 19-year-old cat named Boo, whom I never met in person but sent regular distant treatments. Boo's health had been gradually deteriorating following a stroke-like seizure in 1997. Due to his fragile condition, he wasn't a candidate for any kind of surgery, and it wasn't possible to establish with certainty the exact cause of his problems. He had experienced a short seizure in early 2003, but there was nothing further the vet could do for him. His person was advised that further "neurological events" were likely, and that Boo probably wouldn't survive much longer.

Around this time, after seeing a PBS program about alternative medicine that featured Reiki, Boo's person contacted me to see if Reiki could help him. A distant treatment was tried, and Boo showed noticeable improvement the next day.

Using a stuffed animal as a surrogate, I began offering Boo weekly distant treatments. He was able to live another six months in relative comfort. I learned much from these treatments about his specific health issues. For example, one treatment I gave caused pain in my hand when I did his back right leg. The next day when I spoke by phone to his person, she shared that he had been having weakness in that leg recently. During another treatment, I felt pain in my fingertips when I did his right ear. The person confirmed that he was having difficulty with yeast in that ear. It was quite amazing how powerful distant healing felt not only to Boo, but also to me.

Each time he received a treatment, his person told me that he improved markedly, got a special "glow" and seemed more "there." He slept soundly during the treatments, and never failed to vocalize first thing the next morning with his distinctive sounds of pleasure. Distant Reiki treatment provided a way to significantly improve Boo's quality of life without any of the discomfort and stress involved in taking him out of his familiar surroundings. Although these regular treatments weren't a cure for his health issues, Boo responded so well that his human was inspired to learn Reiki herself so that she could support him with daily treatments. Six months after his first Reiki treatment, Boo peacefully made his transition while at home with his person. —*Kathleen*

into the ebb and flow of the energy and follow your intuition about when the treatment "feels" finished, just as you do with Level 1 Reiki. For example, the dissipation of the flow of energy after it has peaked or your arousal from a deep meditative state can be indicators that the treatment is coming to an end. If you're in the presence of the animal, you can also take note of his behavior, including when he comes out of a relaxed state or when his attention wanders to other matters. A mental healing

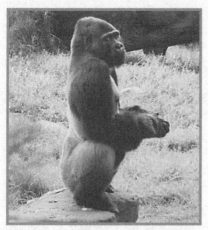
Animals in zoos can greatly benefit from Reiki treatments that are offered from a safe distance.

20 to 30 minutes, or use your intuition to determine when the treatment feels finished.

At the end of a treatment, always say goodbye and thank the animal for being open to the treatment, either in person or mentally if the treatment has been given from far away. Then, just as with Level 1 treatments, thank Reiki for allowing you to be a conduit for the healing process.

is often ending when you feel your inner focus on the treatment lessening or when the energy flow peaks and then, after a few minutes, ebbs to a lower level and remains there. If you're not able to feel the flow of energy yet, you can go by the clock and end the treatment after

As with Level 1 Reiki, it's important to remember that we're merely conduits for the Reiki healing energy, which has its own innate wisdom about what needs to be healed. We don't need to know the source of the problem or its solution; the healing will take place where it's needed most.

chapter 20

Reiki in Shelters, Sanctuaries and Rescue Organizations

WHEN YOU GIVE REIKI TO ANIMALS in shelters, sanctuaries and rescue organizations, the gift will be returned to you a hundred times over in the lessons they teach about healing, love, compassion, forgiveness, trust, patience, resilience and joy. If you're a novice, volunteering in these settings can be a powerful and educational experience and can greatly expand your self-confidence and knowledge of how to heal with Reiki.

By donating your services to a nearby shelter, sanctuary or rescue organization, you'll experience a wide range of the unique situations, issues, challenges and rewards in working with animals in these settings, and these animals can be the best teachers you'll meet in your journey as a healer. The need often seems endless in these places, and you generally can gain as much experience as you wish.

Reiki is a wonderful way to bring hope, healing, relaxation and stress relief to the animals in a shelter, sanctuary or rescue organization. These facilities are filled with wonderful beings who have had difficult journeys in life and are in great need of healing. Working with these animals is very rewarding for both student and animal and quickly builds a beginner's confidence that Reiki can handle a variety of problems effectively. If you have Level 2 Reiki, you can follow up your treatments at a shelter or other organization with distant Reiki for the animal's situation, including issues such as adoption or placement and healing of past trauma and abuse.

Many of these animals have had traumatic experiences involving humans and can benefit tremendously from both the Reiki healing and the association of a human with the experience of being cared about and healed. This is one of the ways in which Reiki can contribute to healing the bond between humans and animals in our world. Reiki practitioners can literally turn lives around in shelter environments and save lives by healing injuries, illnesses and emotional difficulties, such as deep depressions or behavior problems, that would otherwise prevent animals from being adopted. In addition, some of our greatest learning experiences have been with the animals we have encountered in shelters, sanctuaries and rescue organizations.

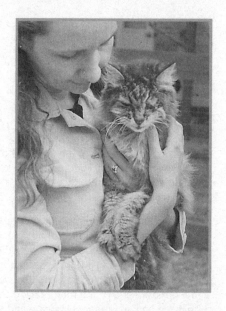

▬ Finding the right place to volunteer

One way to begin the search for a place to volunteer is by compiling a list of appropriate places in your area. These may be city- or county-owned animal shelters, volunteer-run shelters, rescue organizations or animal sanctuaries for small animals (such as cats, rabbits or guinea pigs), horses, farm animals, exotic animals or marine animals. Next, you may want to gather as much information as you can about each organization, such as their mission, their administration, the animals they serve, and volunteer opportunities.

Once you have completed this research, you'll want to visit each of the places that speak strongly to you. You may find that there are one or two that seem an especially good fit for your interests. By visiting the shelter or sanctuary in person, you'll get a feeling for the environment, the animals and the people who work there, so that you can evaluate which places are the best fit for you. Some useful questions to ask yourself are: In which places do I feel most comfortable? Which ones would I enjoy visiting on a regular basis?

Once you've found a couple of places in which you feel comfortable and engaged, you should make an appointment to meet with the volunteer coordinator or the person who runs the organization. This meeting is a good

A MENTAL HEALING FOR MOLLY

Sometimes, a combination of hands-on, mental, distant and situational Reiki is what the animal needs. A perfect example is Molly, a black German shepherd. The first time I worked with her, I gave her a hands-on treatment for an hour. The base of her spine and left hind leg took a lot of Reiki. She was extremely restless and mouthy, scratching up my hands and wrists with her teeth. I kept mentally sending her an image of her mouth being closed and not touching my skin. Finally after 30 minutes, she completely stopped mouthing me. She sat down and turned to face me, putting one front leg over my lap and looking directly at me.

I put one hand on either side of her head in front of her ears, asked permission, and offered her a mental healing, also asking for Divine Order. After a few minutes, I was suddenly hit with the most heartbreaking feeling of sadness that I actually began to cry! I thanked her for sharing with me and let her know I understood. Almost immediately, she moved away from me, sitting at the opposite end of the room, facing the other direction. It was clear to me that she had an emotional release and was "done" with the treatment.

The next week, I learned that Molly had "bitten" (really just mouthed) a volunteer and was being considered for quarantine. I went to visit her in her kennel. When she saw me, she pressed herself up against the wire, looking at me as if to say, "I did a bad thing and I'm in real trouble, but I didn't mean it. I'm sorry." I put a hand through the cage on her back, with my other palm a few inches away outside the cage, and offered Reiki to her. I also sent Reiki for the highest good of her situation, hoping she would find a calm home, away from the stress of the shelter.

Other dogs took precedence for my next few visits to the shelter, but finally a month later, I found myself working with Molly again. I remembered how hyper she was, so I started the treatment from a chair. She was extremely restless, panting and hypervigilant about every noise. She went from door to

way to introduce yourself, describe Reiki, and get a better feel for the organization. We've found that the best approach to describing Reiki is to be as succinct as possible, especially if the person has never heard of it. For example, you can explain that Reiki is a Japanese form of energy healing that is widely used as a comple-

mentary modality for humans, including in many well-known hospitals, and is gaining popularity as a complementary therapy for animals. You can also say that, with Reiki, the practitioner acts as a conduit for the healing energy of the universe to flow through her hands to the animal being treated, healing the animal in the

door, scratching and whining, then back to me, leaning on me so that her left hind leg was off the floor. At one point, a volunteer walked a dog outside the window and Molly went ballistic, barking frantically and looking as if she meant to go through the window to attack the dog.

I decided that distant Reiki was in order. I began to offer the treatment and asked that she be able to receive what she needed despite her state of upset. Amazingly, five to ten minutes later, she lay quietly at my feet. I slowly and carefully lowered myself off the chair and sat at her belly with one hand on her shoulder and the other at the base of her rib cage. She then lay her head on the floor, let out a huge sigh and, incredibly, stopped panting. I continued giving Reiki from this position for 30 minutes. There were some loud noises in the adjacent room, but she didn't even lift her head to look. As I finished the treatment, I put her face between my hands and thanked her. She drowsily looked at me from half-closed eyes, lips loose and hanging. She was a completely different dog: calm, relaxed and trusting. I decided to send several distant treatments that week to help continue her path towards becoming the calm, centered dog that would attract the right loving family.

The next week, I asked to work with Molly again and was told that she was doing so great that she "didn't need it." Smiling, I insisted, and an employee brought her back into the room we used for treatments. This time, when Molly saw me, she immediately lay down and took 45 minutes of Reiki without moving. I gave the entire treatment from the same hand position as the previous week: one hand on her shoulder, the other on her ribs. If I began to move to any other position, she'd start to lift her head and look at me. During the treatment she let out huge sighs and was completely relaxed.

The next time I went to the shelter, Molly wasn't there: she'd found a wonderful home. Apparently, a person absolutely loved her at first sight and seemed to recognize instantly the depth of intelligence and heart that Molly possessed. All the employees were so happy, after all the months of ups and downs, that Molly had found a home. One employee described the adoption as a real "tear jerker." —*Kathleen*

ways that are needed the most. You may want to experiment with your wording until you find a way of talking about Reiki that feels natural and right for you.

Since the person you're meeting may not be familiar with Reiki, it's a good idea to explain in basic terms how Reiki can benefit the organization by helping the animals in their care. For example, you can explain that Reiki will greatly ease the animals' stress and anxiety; it will help them relax in the environment, speed healing of illnesses and injuries, and heal emotional issues that result in behavior problems and impede adoption.

It can help to emphasize that Reiki is extremely gentle and non-invasive, can do no harm, and can be practiced without direct contact with the animal, from outside the kennel or other enclosure or from several feet away from the animal. Sometimes offering to give a short treatment to the person with whom you are speaking will assure them through first-hand experience that Reiki is gentle and comfortable for animals in their care. You could offer to give a short treatment to an animal to demonstrate how Reiki is given. If you have Level 2 Reiki, sending Reiki beforehand to your meeting or conversation about volunteering will help ease the way to a favorable outcome.

Fitting into the organization's environment

Some organizations are overwhelmed with the tasks at hand and will be concerned about the extra work that might be created by your presence. If you let them know that your aim is to be as helpful as possible to the animals without being a burden to the staff, this can be a relief to them and persuade them to give the arrangement a try. You should follow through on your statement by trying to find a way to fit in to the environment with no more assistance from the staff than is necessary.

It's important to remember that you're there to provide Reiki to the animals, not to reorganize and improve the facility or advise the staff. Your goal should be to find a way to fit into the existing environment of the organization, being as unobtrusive, professional, supportive and apolitical as possible. As you develop relationships with some of the employees and volunteers, you may feel comfortable sharing information you receive from your treatments, but it's always best to do so carefully, in a discreet and compassionate way, and without taking sides in organizational matters. If you keep your focus on your work in healing the animals, you will be able to remain there, contributing to their well-being throughout any ups and downs in the organization's operation.

Getting started

Once you've been welcomed into your preferred organization as a Reiki volunteer, it's a good idea to set up a schedule of regular days and times that work well for you and for the organization. If you have other skills that the organization can use, it's better to find different times to perform those tasks and to keep your Reiki time separate.

On the days you arrive for Reiki, you can ask a staff member which animal has the greatest need for healing that day or, if it's acceptable to the organization, you can follow your intuition about which animal or animals need Reiki from you that day. It's best to set aside a 30- to 60-minute block of time for each animal to whom you offer healing. In some organizations, you may be able to find a quiet place in which to give a treatment. If this isn't possible, you can sit inside or just outside the animal's enclosure and offer Reiki. Earplugs can be a great help in focusing on the treatment if the environment is a noisy one.

Offering Reiki to animals in these settings can be stressful as well as rewarding, since there are generally more deserving animals than there is time to offer healing to them all. It's especially important in these settings to be aware of your own internal state and to take care of yourself when you're offering Reiki there. You may want to take particular care to center yourself and give yourself a little Reiki before entering the environment.

It can be important to monitor how much time and effort you spend in these settings and find your own limits so that you don't overextend yourself or draw too heavily on your compassion. Reiki practitioners need to be aware of their limits and should be good to themselves on a regular basis so that they don't burn out and can continue to offer the very best to the animals. Within these parameters, you'll find that the more time you spend volunteering, the more comfortable you'll become giving treatments, the more confident you'll become in Reiki's ability to heal a wide range of challenges effectively, and the more open you'll be to the many lessons the animals have to teach.

chapter 21

Personal Healing and Transformation

IN ADDITION TO ITS USES IN HEALING others, Reiki is a remarkable tool for personal healing and transformation. Reiki can help people as well as animals to resolve and release past memories, patterns, attitudes and other influences that hold them back from the best and highest expression of their true selves. Reiki treatments, especially those including mental and emotional healing, reach deeply into a person or animal's being and bring a profound degree of healing on the emotional and spiritual levels. As you practice Reiki and receive Reiki treatments, it brings out who you are at the most authentic level, enhancing your innate gifts, talents and potential.

While one treatment at times will bring about an extraordinary change, substantial personal transformation generally requires a commitment to regular treatments over an extended period of time. During our training and on an on-going basis throughout our years of practice,

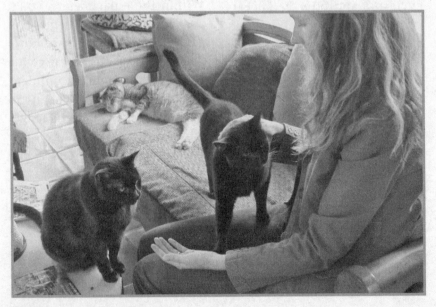

we have continued to treat ourselves daily and to receive weekly or biweekly treatments from others. These treatments maintain our health and enable us to work on personal issues that would otherwise remain obstacles to continued growth in our personal and professional lives.

Becoming a Reiki practitioner is beneficial to your own personal growth as well as others' and, soon after the first attunements, you may begin to notice shifts in your life that coincide with internal healing. At each of the three levels of Reiki, the attunements, along with continued use of Reiki for yourself and others, provide emotional and spiritual healing, accelerated personal growth, and deepened intuition. This accelerated growth can sometimes be challenging (for instance, as old memories and/or patterns are stirred up and released), but its benefits are substantial in terms of personal growth and make the challenges more than worthwhile.

Personal issues can drain our energy, attention and ability to realize our full potential. With Level 2 Reiki, you can send healing to difficult situations in your past to help with the resolution of old difficulties that continue to affect the present. For instance, you can send Reiki to yourself as a child during a particularly difficult time in your life to help resolve any lingering issues related to that time. As you heal your own issues with Reiki, you'll deepen your ability to serve as a conduit for Reiki energy and find that your ability to heal others is strengthened.

In addition to receiving regular treatments from others, we arrange an occasional series of four consecutive treatments to work more intensively on personal issues as the need arises. We treat others, both in person and distantly, as often as possible and continue to offer Reiki treatments as volunteers on a regular basis. We follow up this work with distant treatments for the animals and the organization, and for larger issues that speak to us, such as animal welfare issues, wildlife preservation and the worldwide healing of the human/animal bond. We find that combining these practices on a regular basis accelerates our growth on both the personal and professional levels.

People sometimes ask us why they need to treat themselves or get treatments from others when they only want to heal animals. The answer is that treating yourself and receiving regular treatments from another is central to developing your potential as a healer in two important ways.

First, receiving treatments gives you personal experience with the subtle sensations of receiving Reiki and the process and effects of Reiki healing. This will help you to understand what an animal is feeling during and after a treatment and what kinds of healing and reactions you may expect. It will help you to adjust your treatments to make them more comfortable, acceptable and effective for animals since you'll have first-hand knowledge of the range of sensations and reactions Reiki can involve.

Second, the degree of healing ability that you'll be able to develop is tied to your own personal growth. The more you use Reiki to heal your own issues, the more effective you'll become as a healer. You'll be able to communicate more effectively with the beings you encounter (human and animal), you'll develop increasingly deep and accurate intuition about the beings you treat, and your healing power will increase as you heal personal issues that drain your energy,

ELEPHANTS IN MY PATH

I have always felt a special empathy and connection to shelter and sanctuary animals and harbored an inner desire to help them in any way that I can. Once I became a Reiki Master, there was another way I could help the animals: by teaching Reiki to their caregivers. And once I committed myself to this path, the universe began to open for me in exciting and unexpected ways.

In one particular instance, the animals I was moved to help were elephants. I had by chance caught the nature special, *Urban Elephants*, on PBS. I was so moved by the plight of the world's elephants, I was literally overcome by tears. The show ended, though, on a positive note, by focusing on The Elephant Sanctuary in Tennessee, the only one of its kind in the U.S. It's a place of healing, where elephants are respected, cherished and valued as sentient, spiritual beings. I was especially touched by an amazing reunion of the elephant Shirley with an elephant from whom she had been separated for 25 years.

That night, I decided to do Reiki for the world's elephants. So, using my little wooden Ganesha statue as a surrogate, I cupped my hands, asked permission and asked for highest good and healing for the world's elephants, the ones in the sanctuary (including Shirley), the people running the sanctuary, and how I

attention and ability to tap into your own potential.

The energy attunements combined with self-treatments, receiving treatments and using Reiki to heal others lead to accelerated personal growth, deepened intuition and healing on all levels. The more you use Reiki, the more of these benefits you'll receive, and the more you'll understand the many ways Reiki can heal.

■ Spiritual aspects of Reiki

We sometimes receive questions about whether it's necessary to be religious to use Reiki, whether Reiki itself is a spiritual path, and whether Reiki will interfere with one's religious or spiritual beliefs in any way. Reiki is available as a healing system to anyone who wants to learn it and requires only the attunements from a Reiki Master and some minimal training to get started. It's compatible with any religious tradition, but it isn't necessary to be religious or to follow a spiritual path to practice Reiki. Reiki has spiritual aspects to it on which you can focus if you choose, but this isn't necessary to practice it successfully.

The principles of Reiki are simple and compatible with any religious or spiritual tradition.

might help, if there was a way, with Reiki. The treatment was unusually hot and intense, and didn't seem to let up. After more than an hour, I finished the treatment. My hands were actually in pain: my palms felt like they'd been physically burned and had a sandpaper-like, chafed feeling. I tried to sleep but couldn't. My palms and the soles of my feet were radiating heat all night!

The next day, I decided to see if I could find the sanctuary on the Internet. I found their wonderful website, with stories and pictures of each elephant. I decided to email the founder, even though the website made it clear that they were closed to the public and allowed no visitors. In my email, I offered to teach Reiki to her and her staff, as my gift to the elephants.

That same night, she emailed back and said she rarely allowed people to come, but "sensed" she was "supposed to accept" my gift. A few months later, Elizabeth and I traveled to the sanctuary and taught the founder, co-founder and other full-time employee Level 1 Reiki. We were truly touched and inspired by their love, kindness and dedication to their elephants. They're with the elephants daily, touching them, caring for them, playing with them and feeding them. It's wonderful to know that Reiki is flowing to those wonderful creatures! It's also truly amazing the way Reiki can open the doors to people and places of tremendous healing. (To find out more about The Elephant Sanctuary, visit www.elephants.com.) —*Kathleen*

We know people of many different religious and spiritual backgrounds who practice Reiki with no difficulty with respect to their spiritual beliefs. Reiki can also be practiced solely as a healing system for those who choose not to focus on its spiritual aspects.

For some people, learning and practicing Reiki is a way to feel a stronger connection to spiritual qualities and to psychic energies and abilities. When practiced regularly, Reiki can help you become more aware of your spiritual self, meaning the non-physical inner self, and of subtle gifts and talents that may otherwise go unrealized and untapped. Reiki is complementary to all spiritual paths and religions and can be practiced in a way that reflects the uniqueness of each individual. It also appeals to many people with no spiritual beliefs as a mystery with much empirical evidence to support it.

▬ Personal challenges

As you move forward in your path as an animal Reiki practitioner, you may find yourself encountering new healing challenges in your own life. These challenges may materialize in the form of compelling dreams, sudden realizations about your life's path, the re-emergence of old emotional issues, or coming to terms with unresolved issues from your past. Sometimes old injuries or illnesses that are related to unresolved emotional matters will briefly recur in order to be more thoroughly resolved.

Sometimes the animals themselves will point you in a new direction on your personal path to healing through the emotions and issues that come up around treating them. By using self-treatment and getting regular treatments from another practitioner, you'll be able to use Reiki to guide you through these challenges to greater insights, physical and emotional health, and effectiveness in all areas of your life. The way you use Reiki can be as individual and unique as your own soul. Its essence is pure healing energy and it can only be used for good.

chapter 22

Final Words

From Elizabeth

The visit from the young stag, described in the Preface, began a significant deepening in our understanding of the potential of Reiki. Although I had never met this particular stag before, I had healed other members of the herd in the past, and I had developed close relationships with some of them. But this wasn't one of the individuals I knew well. The possibility that the deer shared with each other their knowledge of where to come for healing was a new and striking development.

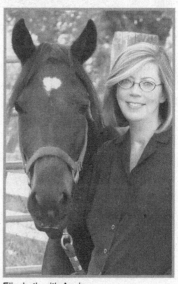
Elizabeth with Annie.

This possibility was confirmed when, several weeks after the young stag had healed, I found a pregnant doe alone in the courtyard with the same purposeful expression that the stag wore when he first arrived for a treatment. By now I knew what it meant and sat down and offered her Reiki. Soon after I began, she stretched her legs out in such a way as to emphasize her belly, as if to say that this was where she wanted the Reiki. From time to time she returned for treatments, and as she approached her delivery date, she began to come more frequently for Reiki. Then, after a few weeks' absence, I was delighted to see her with healthy twin fawns.

From Kathleen

Simultaneously, I began to notice that more and more horses at the barn where I practice Reiki regularly seemed to be asking for Reiki treat-

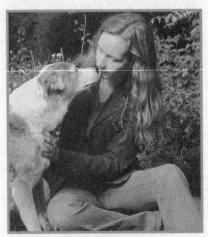
Kathleen bonds with Dakota.

ments. For example, one day as I passed by a paddock of a yearling, a week or two after I had treated a mare in a paddock nearby, the yearling walked quickly and purposefully up to the edge of the paddock so as not to be passed by unnoticed. When I stopped to stroke her head to say hello, the young horse immediately turned her body around and shoved her hip into my hand. The area she placed right under my hands had a deep, painful-looking scrape. Soon after, another horse I wasn't familiar with trotted crookedly up to the fence as I walked. He lifted his hoof purposefully to show me a partially detached shoe that needed immediate attention.

The word is out

When we noticed that more animals were approaching us and asking for healing, it began to dawn on us: "The word is out!" Recognition of the healing energy of Reiki was spreading through the individuals we treated and beyond to other animals in the area. More individuals were coming to trust us to offer this energy to them for healing and to seek it out when they needed it.

Reiki is truly a "frequency" that animals understand and appreciate. The relationship formed between practitioner and animal each time a Reiki treatment is given deepens their understanding of and communication with each other. The connection we have formed with animals through Reiki has transformed our understanding of their natures, cultures and the possibilities within our relationships with them. We believe it has changed their understanding of the possibilities within relationships with humans as well.

Our vision

While working with animals and Reiki, and as the stories throughout this book illustrate, we have realized that in addition to healing individual animals, their humans and situations, Reiki has the potential to heal the connection between humans and animals on a higher level. Increasingly, our vision has expanded to embrace this potential. If other animal lovers learn Reiki and take it out into the world with an open heart, many other animals, domestic and wild, may be drawn to them and come to trust them for healing.

Imagine if many others learned Reiki and, in the process of offering it to the animal kingdom, saw this kind of shift take place in their own relationships with animals. What a profound change could be wrought in the overall relationship between humans and animals in this world! These possibilities further inspire us in our mission.

Our vision is that gradually, through Reiki, individual by individual, human understanding of the nature of animals and the possibilities within the human/ animal relationship will grow and deepen. This deepened understanding may begin with our own animal companions, but as individuals who work or volunteer with animals at marine mammal rescue centers, zoos, wildlife rehabilitation facilities and so on begin to use Reiki with the animals in their care, perhaps human understanding of all of the many different species and our relationships with them will deepen as well.

For those of you who don't already practice Reiki, we hope this book has inspired you to do so. For those of you who are already practitioners, we encourage you to go out with confidence into the world of animal Reiki possibilities. The animals are waiting for us to transform our understanding and fulfill the potential of our relationships with them.

Acknowledgments

With gratitude, first of all, to our wonderful agent, Bobbie Lieberman, who has guided us through the process of a first book with such kindness, patience and expertise, and to our exceptional editors at Ulysses Press, Claire Chun, Lily Chou and Ashley Chase; to Kendra Luck, for capturing the magic of Reiki for animals in her lovely photographs; and to Jamie Westdal and Earl McCowen, for the wonderful photography they also contributed to this book.

With special gratitude and love to my husband, Bob, and daughter, Laura, for all of your patience, love and support throughout the writing process, and to my animal companions, Zoe, Mu Shu, Emma, Smokey, Annie and Senedad, for teaching many of the lessons in this book and inspiring me to do this work and write this book.

I also want to thank Gurumayi Chidvilasananda, for her unfailing Grace and love; Sharon Callahan, whose enormous wisdom and compassion have greatly influenced my understanding of animals and of how to communicate with and heal them; Meg Siddheshwari Sullivan, for the finest education in Reiki; and Tosha Silver, for her invaluable guidance.

Thank you to the City of Berkeley Animal Shelter and the animals who passed through there, and to Carol Buckley and The Elephant Sanctuary.

Thank you to the deer and other wild animals, especially Merlin, who have tutored me patiently and greatly expanded my understanding while inspiring me with their beauty, grace and love; and to my animal and human clients, who continue to enrich my life and my understanding of animals and healing immeasurably.

And finally a heartfelt thank you to my parents, who recognized my bond with animals and enabled me to live closely with animals and nature as a child.

—Elizabeth Fulton

Thank you to my animal companions: my dog, Dakota, and horses, Shawnee and Kodiak. Thank you also to my wonderful animal friends from childhood and youth: our dog, Muffett; our cats, Cassy, Pinky, Jenny, Tux, Anthony and Ginger; my cockatiel, Sherman; my parakeet, Simone; and my goldfish, Sylvia.

Thank you also to my "Reiki animals," precious beings great and small, many still on this planet and many whose spirits have been set free. Meeting and connecting with you, and being able to offer you Reiki and be a part of your journeys has been for me profound and enlightening.

My deepest gratitude and love to my husband, Che, a true Renaissance man: at once logical scientist and physician, creative and diligent musician, and wise and open spiritual soul. You are truly my rock. Thank you to the Prasad family, Judy, Kedar and Mikie. You introduced me to Reiki, and have supported me every step of the way.

A special thanks to my two wonderful sisters, Charlotte and Maureen; you are both truly my best friends. And thank you to my parents, John and Gini, for making my childhood home a place to grow up surrounded by animal friends.

Many thanks and blessings to my Reiki Masters, Martha Lucas and Meg Siddheshwari Sullivan. Thank you also to Tosha Silver, for showing me the way to my inner voice. Blessings to my Reiki students for inspiring me to reach higher.

Big warm hugs to the friends who supported the process: Gail, Susanna, Fray and all of BrightHaven; Alison, my trainer; Emily and PD, Laurel and Picasso, Carol and The Elephant Sanctuary.

Special gratitude to my gifted editor and literary agent, Bobbie Lieberman, and to my talented photographer, Kendra Luck. Your support and belief in this book helped make it become a reality.

—Kathleen Prasad

Appendix

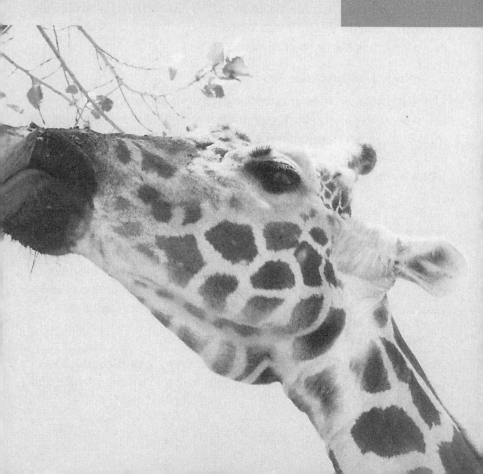

Appendix

■ Resources

www.animalreikisource.com

Animal Reiki Source, founded by coauthor Kathleen Prasad, is the world's first and only nonprofit dedicated to helping rescued animals with Reiki. The site offers an extensive directory of practitioners in the United States as well as Canada, Europe, South America, and Asia.

www.iarp.org

The International Association of Reiki Practitioners has a worldwide directory of Reiki teachers and practitioners. This is a good place to find a Reiki teacher or practitioner.

www.reikialliance.com

The Reiki Alliance is an international community of Reiki Masters of the Usui System of Reiki Healing. They maintain the time-honored form of Reiki passed through the direct lineage of Usui, Hayashi, Takata and Furumoto. This is a good place to find a Reiki teacher or practitioner in the U.S. or abroad.

ANIMAL GROUPS AND SERVICES

www.anaflora.com

Anaflora makes flower essences and essence formulas especially for the challenges that affect animals. Sharon Callahan, the founder of Anaflora, is an internationally recognized animal communicator, and a pioneer in the use of flower essences in the treatment of animals.

www.brighthaven.org

An animal place of love, learning and education, BrightHaven is a non-profit organization dedicated to the well-being of senior, disabled and special animals.

www.elephants.com

The nation's single natural habitat refuge was developed specifically for endangered African and Asian elephants.

www.guidedogs.com

Guide Dogs for the Blind (GDB) provides guide dogs and training for visually impaired people throughout the United States. Its sister organization, Guide Dogs for the Blind International (GDBI), does the same in Canada.

www.naturalhorsetalk.com

Natural Horse Talk educates horse people on using a more natural approach with their horses. For a small fee, users gain access to the site's audio interviews with industry experts.

ANIMAL HOSPICE

www.anaflora.com

This site has an excellent and very moving section ("Grieving the Loss of a Loved Animal") on grieving, the process of death, and what can be done to help a beloved companion facing his transition. See especially the page "When a Beloved Friend Dies or Is Dying."

www.aplb.org

The Association for Pet Loss and Bereavement includes helpful information about euthanasia, a bibliography, a list of support groups, a newsletter and a chat room.

www.blessingthebridge.com

This site accompanies the book of the same name. The author is the founder of an animal sanctuary in Virginia, has established a community animal hospice program, and provides individual consulting. This website also has information about animal hospice, as well as some beautiful stories.

www.in-memory-of-pets.com

This site helps people with the life, love and loss of their animal. After registering for free, you can write in the guestbook, post photos, or submit poems or other written memorials of your beloved animal.

HOLISTIC ANIMAL PUBLICATIONS

www.animalwellnessmagazine.com

This magazine is devoted to educating the public about natural and holistic care options for animals. The company is also focused on helping animals in rescues and shelters; visit rescuenetwork.net for more information and to support these efforts.

www.holistichorse.com

A quarterly publication dedicated to providing information about holistic therapies to equine caretakers, professionals and practitioners of complementary therapies.

www.naturalhorsetalk.com

Natural Horse Magazine focuses on humane and natural care for horses and other animals. There's a relatively low fee that gives you lifetime access to the magazine's hundreds of articles on holistic horse care.

HOLISTIC VETERINARY AND PRACTITIONER DIRECTORIES

www.aava.org

The American Academy of Veterinary Acupuncture's website includes a directory of licensed veterinarians who have completed approved courses in acupuncture and/or traditional Chinese medicine.

www.ahvma.org

The American Holistic Veterinary Medical Association has a directory of holistic veterinarians that practice Reiki and other alternative therapies.

www.alternatives4animals.com

This is a holistic directory of prescreened vets and practitioners trained in alternative and holistic medicine, natural products and animal communicators.

www.avcadoctors.com

The American Veterinary Chiropractic Association's website includes a directory of licensed chiropractors and veterinarians certified in animal chiropractic by AVCA.

www.theavh.org

The Academy of Veterinary Homeopathy's site includes a directory of veterinarians who have been certified as homeopaths by AVH and others who have agreed to practice homeopathy according to the Academy's standards.

REIKI RESEARCH AND INFORMATION

www.nih.gov

The National Institutes of Health, part of the U.S. Department of Health and Human Services, provides government-funded clinical and medical research in a variety of areas. Search "Reiki" for a list of current trials being conducted.

reikiinmedicine.org

Pamela Miles has 30 years of experience as a clinician, educator and lecturer in natural healing. This site offers access to a selection of Reiki-focused medical papers, articles and books.

www.ihreiki.com

This site for The International House of Reiki is a comprehensive resource for information about the system of Reiki.

www.iarp.org

The International Association of Reiki Professionals exists to develop the worldwide Reiki community, to provide a forum for ideas and opinions, and to support all Reiki students and masters.

www.reiki.org

The International Center for Reiki Training offers numerous informational Reiki articles and subscriptions to *Reiki News Magazine*.

■ Recommended Reading

REIKI BOOKS

The Japanese Art of Reiki: A Practical Guide to Self-Healing by Bronwen Stiene and Frans Stiene (Winchester, UK: O Books, 2005)

Reiki by Kajsa Krishni Borang (London, England: Thorsons, 2000). This book has excellent photos of the hand positions for treating people.

The Reiki Handbook: A Manual for Students and Therapists by Larry Arnold and Sandy Nevius (Harrisburg, PA: PSI Press, 1982)

The Reiki Sourcebook by Bronwen Stiene and Frans Stiene (Winchester, UK: O Books, 2003)

Way of Reiki by Kajsa Krishni Borang (London, England: Thorsons, 1997)

Reiki News Magazine

"Reiki at the National Institutes of Health Warren Grant Magnuson Clinical Center" by Pamela Miles. Volume 3, Issue 2, Summer 2004, pp. 52–55.

Radiology Today (this article is available at www.radiologytoday.net):

"Reiki: Rising Star in Complementary Cancer Care" by Kate Jackson. May 12, 2003, pp. 10–13.

Alternative Therapies in Health and Medicine, a peer-reviewed journal (articles are available at www.alternative-therapies.com):

"Reiki Vibrational Healing" by Pamela Miles. Volume 9, Number 4, 2003, pp. 74–83.

"Reiki—Review of a Biofield Therapy: History, Theory, Practice and Research" by Pamela Miles and Gala True. Volume 9, Number 2, 2003, pp. 62–72.

"Preliminary report on the use of Reiki for HIV-related pain and anxiety" by Pamela Miles. Volume 9, Number 2, 2003, p. 36.

"Reiki: A Starting Point for Integrative Medicine" by Robert Schiller, MD. Volume 9, Number 2, 2003, pp. 20–21.

"Enhancing the Treatment of HIV/AIDS with Reiki Training and Treatment" by Robert Schmehr, CSW. Volume 9, Number 2, 2003, p. 120.

ANIMAL HEALTH

Dr. Pitcairn's Complete Guide to Natural Health for Dogs & Cats by Richard H. Pitcairn, DVM, PhD, and Susan Hubble Pitcairn (Emmaus, PA: Rodale Press, 2005)

Four Paws Five Directions: A Guide to Chinese Medicine for Cats and Dogs by Cheryl Schwartz, DVM (Berkeley, CA: Celestial Arts Publications, 1996)

The Goldsteins' Wellness & Longevity Program, Natural Care for Dogs and Cats by Robert S. Goldstein, VMD, and Susan J. Goldstein, TFH (Neptune City, NJ: Publications, Inc., 2005)

The Homoeopathic Treatment of Small Animals: Principles and Practice by Christopher Day, MA, VetMB, VetFFHom, MRCVS (Saffron Waldon, Essex, UK: C.W. Daniel Company, Ltd., 1990)

Natural Healing for Dogs and Cats A-Z by Cheryl Schwartz, DVM (Carlsbad, CA: Hay House, Inc., 2000)

Natural Health Bible for Dogs and Cats: Your A-Z Guide to Over 200 Conditions, Herbs, Vitamins and Supplements by Shawn Messonnier, DVM (Roseville, CA: Prima Publishing, 2001)

Preventing and Treating Cancer in Dogs by Shawn Messonnier, DVM (Novato, CA: New World Library, 2006)

ANIMAL COMMUNICATION

Kinship with All Life by J. Allen Boone (New York: Harper Collins Publishers, 1954)

Reflections of the Heart: What Our Animal Companions Tell Us by Deborah DeMoss Smith (Hoboken, NJ: Wiley Publishing, 2004)

ANIMALS AND SPIRITUALITY

Angel Animals: Exploring Our Spiritual Connection with Animals by Allen and Linda Anderson (New York: The Penguin Group, 1999)

Angel Dogs: Divine Messengers of Love by Allen and Linda Anderson (Novato, CA: New World Library, 2005)

Animal Grace: Entering a Spiritual Relationship with Our Fellow Creatures by Mary Lou Randour (Novato, CA: New World Library, 2000)

Animal Passions and Beastly Virtues: Reflections on Redecorating Nature by Marc Bekoff (Philadelphia, PA: Temple University Press, 2005)

Animals as Guides for the Soul by Susan Chernak McElroy (New York: Ballantine Publishing Group, 1998)

Animals as Teachers and Healers by Susan Chernak McElroy (New York: Ballantine Publishing Group, 1996)

"The Care and Feeding of an Animal Soul" by Sharon Callahan at www.anaflora.com.

Chicken Soup for the Pet Lover's Soul by Jack Canfield, Marty Becker, DVM, et al. (Deerfield Beach, FL: HCI, 1998)

Dogs Never Lie about Love: Reflections on the Emotional World of Dogs by Jeffrey Moussaieff Masson (New York: Crown, 1997)

The Encyclopedia of Animal Behavior by Marc Bekoff (Westport, CT: Greenwood Press, 2004)

God's Messengers: What Animals Teach Us about the Divine by Allen and Linda Anderson (Novato, CA: New World Library, 2003)

Heart in the Wild: A Journey of Self-Discovery with Animals of the Wilderness by Susan Chernak Mcelroy (New York: The Ballantine Publishing Group, 2002)

If You Tame Me: Understanding Our Connection with Animals (Animals, Culture and Society) by Marc Bekoff (Philadelphia, PA: Temple University Press, 2004)

Minding Animals: Awareness, Emotions and Heart by Marc Bekoff, Jane Goodall (New York: Oxford University Press, 2002)

Reason for Hope: A Spiritual Journey by Jane Goodall with Phillip Berman (New York: Warner Books, 1999)

Reflections of the Heart: What Our Animal Companions Tell Us by Deborah DeMoss Smith (Hoboken, NJ: Wiley Publishing, 2004)

She Flies without Wings: How Horses Touch a Woman's Soul by Mary D. Midkiff (New York: Random House, 2001)

The Smile of a Dolphin: Remarkable Accounts of Animal Emotion by Marc Bekoff, ed. (New York: Discovery Books/Random House, 2000)

Strolling with Our Kin: Speaking for and Respecting Voiceless Animals by Marc Bekoff (Jenkintown, PA: American Anti-Vivisection Society, 2000)

The Tao of Equus by Linda Kohanov (Novato, CA: New World Library, 2001)

The Ten Trusts: What We Must Do to Care for the Animals We Love by Jane Goodall and Marc Bekoff (New York: Harper Collins Publishers, Inc., 2002)

When Elephants Weep: The Emotional Lives of Animals by Jeffrey Moussaieff Masson and Susan McCarthy (New York: Dell Publishing, 1995)

The Wild Parrots of Telegraph Hill: A Love Story . . . with Wings by Mark Bittner (New York: Three Rivers Press, 2005)

DEATH AND DYING/HOSPICE CARE

Animals and the Afterlife by Kim Sheridan (Escondido, CA: EnLighthouse Publishing, 2003)

Blessing the Bridge: What Animals Teach Us about Death, Dying and Beyond by Rita Reynolds (Troutdale, OR: NewSage Press, 2001)

On Death and Dying by Elisabeth Kubler-Ross, MD (New York: Simon & Schuster, 1969)

The Tibetan Book of Living and Dying by Sogyal Rinpoche (New York: Harper Collins Publishers, 2002)

The Tunnel and the Light by Elisabeth Kubler-Ross, MD (New York: Marlow & Co., 1999)

FLOWER ESSENCES

The Bach Flower Remedies Step by Step by Judy Howard (Saffron Waldon, Essex, UK: C.W Daniel Company, Ltd., 1990)

The Bach Remedy Newsletter, issued by the Bach Centre three times a year. Available through Dr. Edward Bach Centre, Mount Vernon, Sotwell, Wallingford, Oxon OX10 OPZ, United Kingdom; phone (44) 01491 834678

Healing Animals Naturally with Flower Essences and Intuitive Listening by Sharon Callahan (Mt. Shasta, CA: Sacred Spirit Publishing, 2001)

Seven Herbs: Plants as Teachers by Matthew Wood (Berkeley, CA: North Atlantic Books & Homeopathic Education Service, 1986)

The Twelve Healers and Other Remedies by Edward Bach (Woodstock, NY: Beekman Publishers, Inc., 1999)

Index

BrightHaven

We could not have done this book without the generosity of the staff and animals of BrightHaven. This California non-profit organization provides lifetime sanctuary and hospice care to senior, disabled and special-needs animals. Ollie, Ted, Harley, Dorothy and Frazier, all models in this book, call BrightHaven home.

Since its inception in the early 1990s, BrightHaven has rescued and cared for countless unadoptable animals. Cats and dogs spend their golden years in a loving family environment where they are cared for naturally, including a raw meat diet and holistic health care. BrightHaven has seen many miracles resulting from its balance of love, healthy diet and healing art forms such as Reiki and homeopathy.

After more than a decade of learning about the best ways to care for animals, BrightHaven has opened its doors to share its vast experience through an innovative program of workshops and seminars. Tax-deductible donations are welcome, and will help BrightHaven continue its important work.

For further information, please visit www.brighthaven.org or call the BrightHaven office at (760) 423-6262.

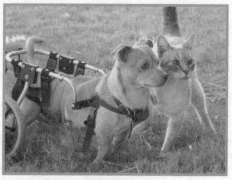

Joey the dog enjoys a moment with Oliver.

Other Books from Ulysses Press

REIKI FOR DOGS: USING SPIRITUAL ENERGY TO HEAL AND VITALIZE MAN'S BEST FRIEND
Kathleen Prasad, $14.95
Shows how anyone can help heal their dog using "hands-on" Reiki therapies.

COLORING ANIMAL MANDALAS
Wendy Piersall, $10.00
Attain focus, clarity, and peace while adding bright and inspiring colors to these unique patterns.

DAILY ZEN DOODLES: 365 TANGLE CREATIONS FOR INSPIRATION, RELAXATION AND JOY
Meera Lee Patel, $16.95
A year's worth of "tangled drawings" designed to inspire creativity and serenity.

To order these books call 800-377-2542 or 510-601-8301, fax 510-601-8307, e-mail ulysses@ulyssespress.com, or write to Ulysses Press, P.O. Box 3440, Berkeley, CA 94703. All retail orders are shipped free of charge. California residents must include sales tax. Allow two to three weeks for delivery.

About the Authors

Elizabeth Fulton is an animal communicator, Reiki Master and founder of the Animal Healing Institute, dedicated to the deep healing of animals and of our bond with them. She was one of the first people to offer Reiki professionally to animals. Using animal communication, Reiki and flower essences, she assists animals and their people in understanding each other and healing the physical, emotional and spiritual challenges that arise in their lives. Elizabeth writes about animal communication and healing and the potential of our relationships with animals. She donates her services to several sanctuaries and other organizations oriented toward wild, exotic and endangered animals. Visit Elizabeth online at www.healingforanimals.com.

Kathleen Prasad is founder and director of Animal Reiki Source in San Rafael, California, which is dedicated to educating the public about Reiki for animals through treatments, training programs, speaking engagements, publications and research. She has been a Reiki practitioner since 1998 and a Reiki Master since 2001. Initially learning Reiki as a tool for self-healing, Kathleen rapidly discovered that animals of all species were drawn to the healing power of Reiki. Her lifelong love for animals' inspired her to provide programs to empower people to help the animals in their lives. She encourages the use of Reiki in shelters, rescue organizations and sanctuaries, donating her services regularly. Visit Kathleen online at www.animalreikisource.com.

Dr. Cheryl Schwartz, the author of the foreword, has been a practicing veterinarian for more than 25 years. She specializes in the use of Chinese medical diagnosis, acupuncture and Chinese herbs for small animals. A pioneer in introducing holistic medicine to the veterinary field, she founded the East-West Animal Care Center, which trained veterinarians in Chinese medicine. Dr. Schwartz is also author of *Four Paws, Five Directions: A Guide to Chinese Medicine for Cats & Dogs* and a holistic pet care columnist for *Healthy Living Magazine*.